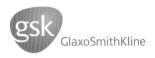

The expression "a picture is worth a thousand words" is particularly appropriate when it refers to medical photographs. Words alone can never create the profound impact of photographs that vividly illustrate diseases a physician might still encounter, as well as those that have already been brought under control.

Today, we no longer consider epidemics of the past as public threats. Yet, with ever-changing global dynamics, physicians must be prepared for the possible return of past scourges. An example is smallpox - shocking but possibly real because of today's new and frightening threats. President Bush recently announced that to protect Americans, the smallpox vaccine will be made available, beginning with the military and health care workers. But preparation begins in many ways, including an understanding and recognition of the physical, mental, and social impact these diseases once had on the population. Medical photography can help us reach that understanding.

GlaxoSmithKline, in its continual effort to serve the public welfare and the medical community, has commissioned an original educational series of four photographic books on the history of medicine from the Burns Archive of Medical Photographic History. These original works, titled "Respiratory Disease: A Photographic History 1845 to 1945," will encourage physicians to think about past medical practices and how medicine has progressed over its most critical century.

This collection, by renowned physician and historian Stanley B. Burns, dominates the field of early medical photography, containing more than 50,000 medically significant photographs. Many of them, complete with written explanations, have never been seen by the general medical profession.

Dr. Burns has published more than a dozen books and his collection has been the subject of numerous exhibitions. Recent presentations have been mounted at the Musee d'Orsay, Paris; Kulturbro 2002 Art Biennial, Brosarp, Sweden; The Center for The Study of the United States, Haifa, Israel; and the National Arts Club, New York. Dr. Burns' full collection of over 700,000 photographs are used by researchers, book publishers, media and film companies worldwide.

GSK is proud to sponsor this original Historical Medical Educational Series.

Chris Viehbacher
President, US Pharmaceuticals
GlaxoSmithKline

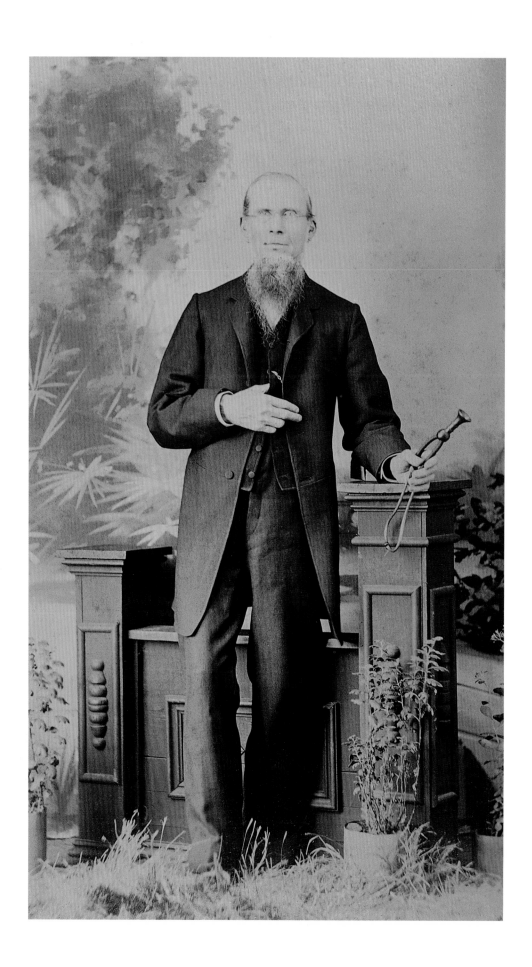

RESPIRATORY DISEASE:

A PHOTOGRAPHIC HISTORY
1845-1870 THE PIONEER ERA
SELECTIONS FROM *THE BURNS ARCHIVE*

STANLEY B. BURNS, M.D.

BURNS ARCHIVE PRESS
NEW YORK 2003

Colophon

This first edition of *Respiratory Disease: A Photographic History, 1845-1870 The Pioneer Era* is limited to 20,150 copies including a special cased edition of 1000 copies. The photographs are copyright Stanley B. Burns, MD & The Burns Archive. The design is copyright Elizabeth A. Burns & The Burns Archive. The text and contents of this volume are copyright Stanley B. Burns, MD, 2003. Printed and bound in China for The Burns Archive Press, NY, a division of Burns Archive Photographic Distributors, Ltd. NY. The book is printed on acid free 140 GMS Hi-Q Matte paper. The 4-color separations were scanned at 200 lines per square inch.

ISBN: 0-9612958-4-8

Library of Congress Cataloging-in-Publication Data:
Burns, Stanley B.
Respiratory Disease: A Photographic History: 1845-1870 The Pioneer Era
    Includes bibliographical references: 1. Medical, History 2. Respiratory Disease
    3. Photography, History 4. Civil War 5. Lung Disease 6. Infectious Disease
    7. Medical Instruments 8. Stanley B. Burns, MD

The Burns Archive Press

Author & Publisher: Stanley B. Burns, MD
Editor: Sara Cleary-Burns
Production & Design: Elizabeth A. Burns

Photographic Captions

Front Cover: Physician Posing with Laënnec Model Stethoscope, Carte de Visite, 1860
In 1819 and again in 1826, French internist, Rene T. H. Laënnec (1781-1826), changed the nature of medical practice with both his invention of the stethoscope and the publication of two volumes on diagnosing chest disease. These books formed the foundation of modern knowledge of chest disease and diagnosis by auscultation. The original instrument was a simple hollow, wooden tube. To this day the stethoscope remains the basic tool of the chest physician continues to be improved. The instrument not only enhanced audible chest sounds but created another major advantage as the physician could examine the contagious patient from a safe distance rather than having to put his ear against his chest. This physician is posing with an advanced model of the single tube Laënnec stethoscope.

Frontispiece: Physician with a Binaural Stethoscope, Cabinet Card, 1870
The practical binaural stethoscope was America's contribution to the advancement in the diagnosis of chest disease. By the mid-1880s, American physicians had turned toward the binaural scope. While it was a better auditory tool than the simple monaural scope, the monaural scope remained popular in Europe until well into the twentieth century. This American physician casually poses with his instrument.

Back Cover: Viennese Otolaryngologist Posing with Her Instruments, Carte de Visite, 1870
This physician poses with the tools of a pioneer laryngologist. A head mirror lies on the table along with mirrors to examine the larynx and nasal passages. The curved probe in her hand was probably used to remove or move tissue.

Contents

PREFACE

As an ophthalmologist, a life-long collector and a historian, I am fascinated by our past and drawn to visualizing history. When I first started collecting medical photographs in 1975, I chose images based on both their importance as historic documents and as evidence of medicine's rich past. What I soon realized was their artistic strength.

In 1979, I created the Burns Archive, which is dedicated to preserving medical photographs and producing publications on the history of medical photography. By the mid-1980s, noted curators and artists became interested in medical photography as art. Marvin Heiferman curated "In the Picture of Health" in 1984, an exhibit of more than 140 photographs from the Archive. This was the first exhibition of medical photographs in a public art institution. In 1987, Joel-Peter Witkin edited *Masterpieces of Photography: Selections from the Burns Archive*. Since then, numerous major museums and galleries, recognizing the artistic value of these images, have started to collect and exhibit medical photography. These institutions now display vintage medical photographs of patients, procedures and practitioners to the general public.

What I have learned these past twenty-eight years is that art matters. Art elevates and stimulates us to see things differently. Art creates a different perspective and point of view. When medical photographs are presented to the public, the images are viewed and conceived in terms of personal mortality, human fragility and the vagaries of life. Terror and fascination draw the non-medical public into dialogue with these images. Although the art world's appreciation of vintage medical photography as art is laudable, my original goal as a historian was to present these photographs to my colleagues not as art, but as historic documents. I want my fellow physicians to visually experience the practice of medicine in the 19th century to help them gain a better understanding of the foundation of our therapies and patient treatment. As a physician, I am brought back to a different reality by these photographs. I see my patients; I see difficulties in therapy, I see personal challenges and I wonder whether what I am doing and what I believe in will one day be proven wrong.

GlaxoSmithKline has given me the opportunity to share with my colleagues these photographs on respiratory disease. This compilation is not meant to be an encyclopedic history of the topic, but to put the emphasis on artistic, medical photographs that will allow you to see the transition of medicine from yesterday to today. Many of the treatments depicted have long since become outmoded, but our predecessors believed they were offering the best therapy available. My hope is that you will look at these images as icons of our past and gain a better understanding of what we do and how we can better serve our patients.

Medicine's quest to unselfishly help and heal is one of mankind's highest goals. I am proud to be part of the medical profession and share these photographs to further that goal.

Stanley B. Burns, M.D., F.A.C.S.
New York, March 2003

INTRODUCTION

This is the first photographic work documenting respiratory tract disease and its impact on the practice of medicine. The rare photographs in this compilation are from private albums and sources now in the Burns Archive. Many are either published here for the first time or have not been published since their original presentation. The book begins with the earliest known photographs related to respiratory tract disease. It ends in 1945, at the close of World War II, when penicillin and other antibiotics became generally available and put an end to thousands of years of deadly respiratory tract infections. In the pre-antibiotic era, especially in the nineteenth century, infectious disease ran rampant and physicians often did as much harm as good. The photographs in this book are true 'history,' not 'heritage.' Heritage is the daydream of history, that part we want to remember. Heritage is a pick-and-choose process so that it seems there is an unbroken line of good choices leading to current philosophies. In medicine, that is often far from the truth. History is the whole picture, the good with the bad. Much of medical photographic history has been lost because few want to preserve the evidence of poor treatment or erroneous theories. Fortunately, some photographs have survived and this book provides a unique glimpse through a window in time of our predecessors, their patients and their tribulations.

Modern Medicine and the Respiratory Tract

Modern medicine was born through the respiratory tract! In 1819, Dr. Rene Laënnec invented the first modern diagnostic instrument, the stethoscope. It has become a symbol of medicine, an icon of the profession. Through the use of gas in the treatment of respiratory disease in the 1840s, health care professionals were fortunate to discover the anesthetizing effects of nitrous oxide and sulfuric ether. The year 1846 marks the beginning of the modern medical era with the introduction of anesthesia, the first of modern medicine's miracles. With the invention of two other major medical tools to examine respiratory tract organs, the laryngoscope in 1854, and the otoscope in 1860, the medical specialty of otorhinolaryngology was founded. The nose, throat and the ears, integral parts of the respiratory system, are often involved in respiratory system disease.

Investigation of respiratory tract disease provided physicians with modern medicine's basic tools to find the cause of disease and the first specific therapy. Dr. Robert Koch discovered the bacterial cause of tuberculosis and established the principles of the germ theory of disease in 1882. His postulates for establishing the etiology of a disease are followed to this day . They are the basis of modern bacteriology concepts. The laboratories and research became the backbone of medicine. In 1890, Dr. Emil von Behring discovered the first specific medical therapy, diphtheria antitoxin. Improved sanitation and public health measures instituted at the turn of the century resulted in a further decrease of respiratory disease.

The first third of the twentieth century witnessed research in anti-serum and vaccine development as the main thrust of medical therapeutic and immunologic science. Technological advances, many using photography as a base, allowed the development of sophisticated tools to treat and diagnose disease. Photography played a major role in this advancement. The X-ray, camera, television, computers and other photographically based imaging devices were an essential aspect of many of these devices. Endoscopic imaging and the TV monitor provide the latest in twenty-first century diagnostic and surgical procedures.

Respiratory Tract Disease

It must be noted that respiratory tract disease was the number one killer in the nineteenth and early twentieth centuries. Of these, tuberculosis was the most feared, nicknamed "The Captain of All the Men of Death." Many of those who did not die from the disease were disfigured and disabled for life. Diphtheria and scarlet fever, infections of the respiratory tract, caused the deaths of uncountable numbers of children. Combined with pneumonia, influenza and pneumonic plague, respiratory diseases reigned for centuries. It is no wonder that medical science directed its attention to the control of respiratory tract diseases. With the advent of antibiotics and chemotherapy, infectious respiratory disease was essentially conquered. However, modern cities, with their increased industrial pollution, have created serious new respiratory conditions. Asthma and allergies have become a focus of concern. Treatment of respiratory based gaseous and chemical weapons is another contemporary medical issue and research focus.

Photography in Medicine

Photography was presented to the world in 1839 and its use was immediately adopted by physicians to document unusual cases, portraits of medical pioneers, and the everyday practitioners of medicine. The compilation of photographs within this book reflects medicine's preoccupation with respiratory tract disease. It is not only a history of the major achievements, however, but emphasizes the struggle of physicians and their patients. In addition to presenting the images of professional photographers, the book includes vernacular photographs, those taken by, of, or for physicians. These photographs follow the changing nature of the practice of medicine. They are a testament to the effort of the health care practitioners to heal and comfort their patients in an era of medical ignorance.

Photographs can serve not only to reveal the challenges met by our predecessors but as visual tools for the modern practitioner to contemplate his or her own work. When viewing a photograph of the whole patient along with his disease, one is forced to confront the patient as a person. Modern medical practice has been criticized as not being holistic in its approach, as treating diseases, not patients. These images help create a special empathy and concern for the patient. While the general public may look at these pictures with terror and fascination, physicians can come closer to understanding the problems. They are not repulsed but are drawn to the patient by the well-known phenomena of "magical substitution," or, simply stated, by placing themselves mentally into the photograph. Physicians often take pause and contemplate their own therapies as they recognize that the treatment shown in the photograph was thought to be the latest and best, though time proved many to be deleterious or, at best, erroneous.

THE PIONEER ERA 1845-1870

During the years 1845-1870 two of the four major medical advances of the nineteenth century took place. In 1846, general anesthesia was discovered and in 1867, Sir Joseph Lister presented his concepts on antiseptic wound healing, based on the research of Louis Pasteur. The ophthalmoscope (1851), laryngoscope (1854), and otoscope (1860) were also invented. The use of these instruments helped create medical specialties. The American binaural stethoscope (1855) advanced the diagnosis technique for chest disease. During the nineteenth century respiratory tract disease was the number one killer of both adults and children. Photography, perfected in 1840, was available to record these triumphs and their effect on the practice of medicine. The Civil War was the defining event of this era. This book presents for the first time a visual study of chest wounds from this war. Photographs of practitioners and patients with extremes of disease complete this volume.

1
Pneumatologists and Respiratory Disease Treatment
Stereoview
circa 1855

This amusing photograph of gas inhalation represents a critical stage in the histories of both respiratory disease treatment and general anesthesia. There are no other known early photographs of this gas inhalation phenomenon.

The inhalation of various gasses as, treatment for respiratory disease and social entertainment, became popular in the eighteenth century. In 1772, Joseph Priestly (1733-1804), the noted chemist and a pioneer in physiology, isolated not only oxygen, but nitrous oxide commonly known as laughing gas. In his *Experiments and Observations Concerning the Different Kinds of Air*, he attempted to explain the nature of gas exchanges in the lungs. His conclusions were close but in inverted order. It remained for the French chemist, Antoine Laurent Lavoisier (1743-1794), father of modern chemistry, to clearly explain the modern theory of respiration. Lavoisier delineated the composition of the gases of respiration and the true nature of the gaseous exchange in the body. The importance of oxygen, nitrogen, carbon dioxide exchange was documented. Unfortunately, he was beheaded during the French revolution.

With the elucidation of the importance of various gases, especially oxygen in respiration, physicians were carried away in their fervor to attribute disease to either an excess, lack of oxygen, or, perhaps, some other gaseous substance in the air. These physicians. 'pneumatologists', established a specialty in pneumatic medicine. They treated disease by gas administration. Oxygen was the favored gas, however, noxious gases were also popular, especially chlorine. This gas remained in use to treat colds until almost the mid-twentieth century. Asthma, catarrh, tuberculosis and all breathing difficulties were treated with various gases. As with all new branches of medicine the pneumatologists soon extended their methods to include treatments of cancer, psychiatric, neurological and other diseases. In this early era of no specific therapies these respiratory treatment seemed as good as any. The new gas treatments were promoted as 'the elixir of life'. A century later electric treatments would be similarly heralded as a 'cure all' noting that electricity was the basic physiologic phenomena.

The most heralded pneumatologist was Dr. Thomas Beddoes (1760-1808). He established *The Pneumatic Institute* located in Clifton, near Bristol, England. In 1799, his assistant, the English scientist, Humphrey Davy, introduced nitric oxide gas to pneumatic therapy and suggested its use for pain relief during surgery. Sadly his medical colleagues refused to take the anesthesia possibilities seriously. Over the next 50 years scientists would isolate numerous other gases that have had a profound effect in medicine. In 1831, three scientists working independently discovered chloroform. Ether and nitrous oxide were found to have a euphoric effect and soon ether frolics or parties were part of the 1830s social scene. At these parties some would fall and hurt themselves but felt no pain. The lack of pain in those individuals lead innovative minds to eventually use the substance for general anesthesia. The inhalation of ether, chloroform, nitrous oxide, chlorine, oxygen and other gases remained part of pneumatic medicine for much of the nineteenth century. Although Dr. Beddoes' idea of respiratory treatment by gases fell into general disfavor it was revived in the twentieth century when the inhalation of various gases became standard practice. Two of these treatments were aerotherapy or pneumotherapy as they were called in the mid-twentieth century. The atmospheric oxygen tent was also an innovation that saved countless lives. Today a respiratory therapist is an active part of the medical team.

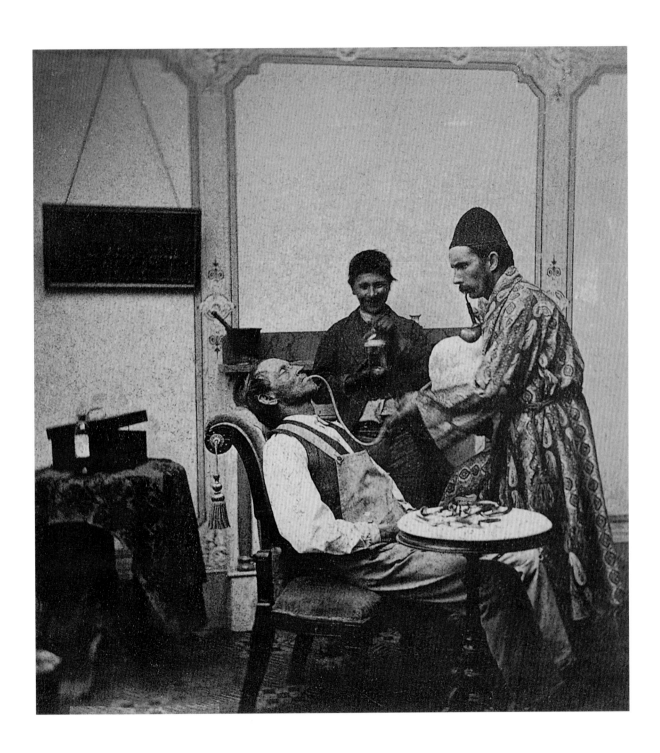

2
DOCTOR POSING WITH HIS OPERATIVE INSTRUMENTS
DAGUERREOTYPE
CIRCA 1845

Painted portraits had long been one of the only ways to capture the likeness of a loved one, event or person of importance. However, the cost of a painting was well over what the middle or working class individual could afford. Photography brought democracy to the world of portraiture. As photography developed several special styles of poses emerged. By the early 1840s, the convention of photographing people with the tools of their trade became popular and it remained popular for over 30 years. Occupations were, and often still are, the defining characteristic of one's life. A photographic portrait taken in photography's early years was still relatively expensive and for many a once-in-a-lifetime event. Physicians chose to pose with three main props; a skull, books or medical instruments. Each represented or symbolized the special status held in society by the physician. The skull represented knowledge of life and death; books illustrated a professional education; and instruments showed the competence to operate and treat the patient. As photography advanced the photograph was used as an advertising tool and physicians depicted themselves with the latest medical equipment. This style is used to this day as physicians pose next to lasers, ultrasound machines or other specialized instruments. This photograph of a physician posing with his medical kit is a daguerreotype, the earliest form of photography, and represents the beginning of photographic, occupational portraiture.

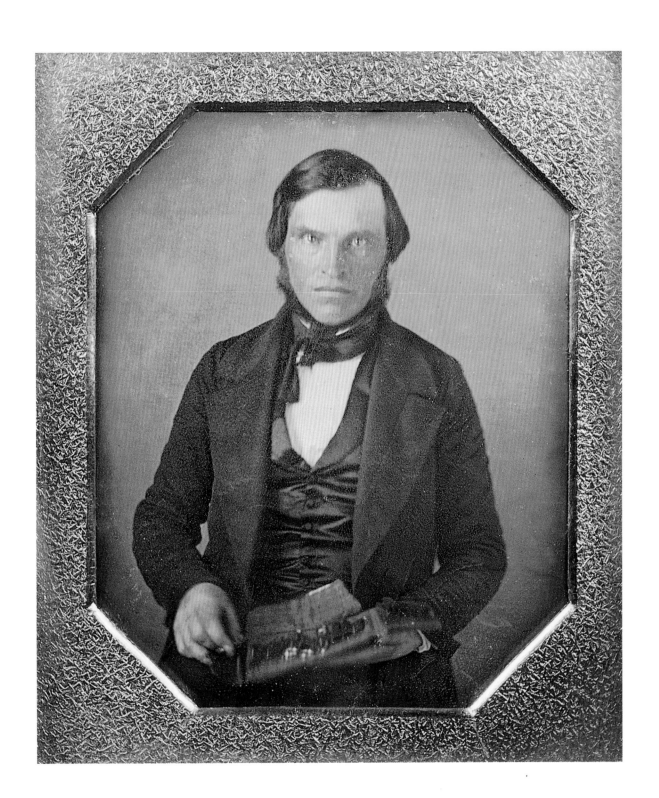

3
EARLY GENERAL ANESTHESIA OPERATION
MASSACHUSETTS GENERAL HOSPITAL
DAGUERREOTYPE
BOSTON, MASSACHUSETTS
WINTER 1846/7

The general anesthetic effects of both ether and nitrous oxide were ultimately discovered by the use of gas in respiratory therapy. On October 16, 1846, the first surgical procedure and public demonstration of the anesthetic effects of sulfuric ether was performed. Photographer, Josiah H. Hawes, was present and ready to record the event but he was so unnerved by the sight of blood that he did not take the photograph. In this later daguerreotype by Hawes, ten physicians, including Chief Surgeon, John Collins Warren, M.D., (1778-1856), look up at the camera. William T.G. Morton (1819-1868), the Boston dentist who first demonstrated sulfuric ether, was not a member of this surgical team.

Three men were associated with the attempt in Boston to bring anesthetic effects into general use. Dentist Horace Wells (1815-1848), recognized nitrous oxide's ability to produce anesthesia. In 1844 he tried to use it in a public demonstration at Massachusetts General Hospital. The demonstration failed. Thomas Charles Jackson (1805-1880), a chemist, suggested the use of sulfuric ether as an anesthetic to dentist William T.G. Morton. Morton was successful in his demonstration, but, unfortunately, he was greedy and attempted to keep the gas a secret. He named it 'Letheon' and hoped to secure a patent. He did not mention Jackson's critical role in its use. All of the pioneers involved in the development of anesthesia use at Massachusetts Hospital, Morton, Jackson and Wells, fought for rights to primacy of the discovery. They all died poor and in dire circumstances. Morton died at age 49 on July 15, 1868 in New York's Central Park. He suffered a stroke after reading a magazine report supporting Well's claim. Jackson spent his life fighting the findings of the U.S. government and others that Morton was the sole inventor. He went insane in Boston's Mt. Auburn Cemetery after reading Morton's monument describing him as the inventor. Jackson spent the rest of his years, often in restraints, at McLean Asylum in Somerville. He died there August 28, 1880. Horace Wells also had a tragic ending. Not achieving his due credit for his work in the promotion of anesthesia he too went insane. He was arrested for throwing ether on women in New York City and committed suicide in his jail cell. Ironically another physician was given the credit for being the first to use sulfuric ether as an anesthetic, Crawford Williamson Long, M.D. (1815-1878). A country doctor from Jefferson, Georgia, Long first used ether in March of 1842 and continued its use. However, as he was out of the academic circle and perhaps did not fully appreciate his discovery, he did not publish his results until 1849. Several of Long's early operations were witnessed by other physicians and their affidavits backed his claim. Long had gotten the idea in the winter of 1841 when some chemistry students who had participated in nitrous oxide parties asked Long to prepare nitrous oxide for them. Long didn't know how to make nitrous oxide but knew how to make sulfuric ether. This gas was supposed to have a similar physical effect upon inhalation. At the party Long noticed the men having hilarious fun were bruised by falls and yet felt no pain. On this basis Dr. Long reasoned the gas must have an anesthetic effect and proposed using it in surgery.

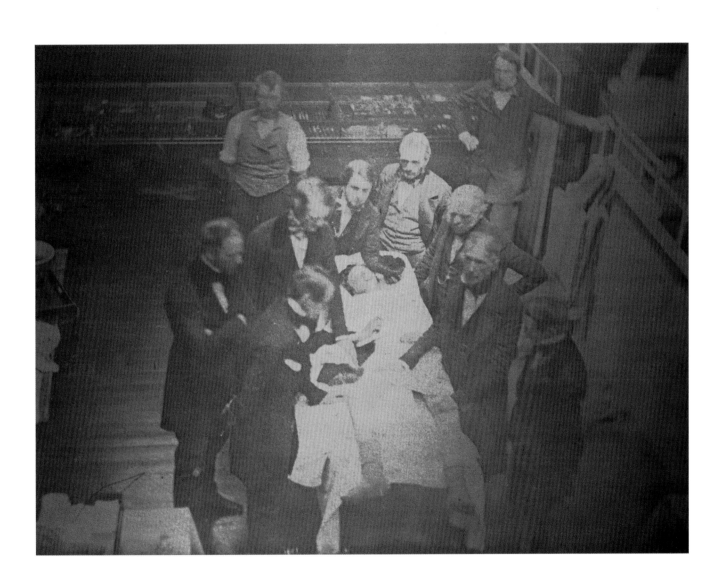

4
A Mother with Her Dead Daughter
Post Mortem Photograph
Daguerreotype
circa 1854

In photography's earliest era, most middle and working class people could not afford to have a photograph taken or did not have easy access to a photographer. The expense could not be justified during one's lifetime, but at death it was the only way to preserve the visual memory. Until the second decade of the twentieth century taking a photograph of a deceased loved one was a normal part of American culture. It was very common to see a parent posed with their dead child or a sibling posed with their dead brother or sister. These photographs documented their family bonds. Today many hospitals advocate the taking of a postmortem photograph of babies stillborn or neo-natal deaths so the parents can have a visual record of the child. Some pose with the child in the nineteenth century convention. These post mortem photographs have been found to be an important psychological aid in the bereavement process. This post mortem photograph clearly shows a healthy looking young girl. In the nineteenth century childhood diseases, especially respiratory diseases, killed quickly. A family could lose all of their children in a matter of days. Diphtheria and scarlet fever caused virulent epidemics and was the scourge of childhood. Death by intestinal disease was also common in the very young and photographs depict those children usually with visible dehydration.

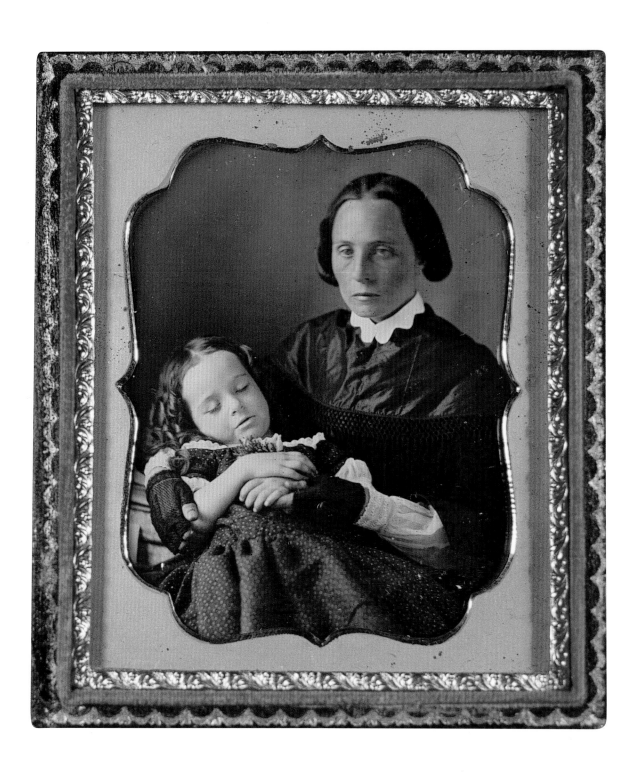

SNUFFING & TOBACCOSIS:
THE FOREMOST PLAGUE OF THE TWENTIETH CENTURY

AMBROTYPE
CIRCA 1855

The respiratory system was used as a portal of entry for a variety of medications including various gases, steamed vapors, chemical and organic inhalants. Tobacco was among the most powerful inhalants.

Physicians have considered tobacco a potent medicinal since its introduction into Western culture. For centuries the American Indians used tobacco for ceremonial, medicinal and intoxicating effects. Columbus brought tobacco to Western Europe. Pipe smoking was the most common method of consumption. In the 1700s, the European upper classes began the practice of snuffing tobacco dust. Snuff is a pure tobacco product made by crushing the cured leaves into a powder. It has one of the highest nicotine contents and, like cocaine and other inhalants, not only is it absorbed into the body through the lungs, it goes directly to the bloodstream through the mucus membranes of the nose and throat. The first clinical report of cancer due to tobacco use appeared in 1761. John Hill, M.D., an English physician, documented with a detailed description the progress of nose cancer developed by a snuff user. Percival Pott, M.D. (1744-1788), London's most distinguished surgeon of the era, reported in 1775 on the frequent occurrence of scrotal cancer in chimney sweeps. He ascribed the disease to the carcinogenic effect of chimney smoke. Until the end of the nineteenth century when laboratory diagnosis became established, lung cancer was often lumped together with other lung diseases into the wastebasket terms of phthisis or consumption.

Full strength tobacco was used as a treatment for numerous diseases via inhalation or snuff. It was also a component in many of the allopathic medicines, salves, suppositories, elixirs, pills, lotions and injections. By the end of the nineteenth century tobacco was available in numerous forms for recreational use. Cigarettes were introduced in America from England mid-century and became increasingly popular. By 1880, about 1.3 billion cigarettes were consumed annually. Smoking tobacco leaves rolled into cigars were available. Lip and oral cancers were recognized by astute physicians as being caused by cigar and other oral tobacco products such as chewing tobacco, a mixture of tobacco and molasses. Chewing tobacco was the leading form of tobacco consumption in the United States. Physicians began to note the occurrence of respiratory system cancers and by the 1880s warnings against tobacco use began to appear.

Tobaccosis is a term coined by R.T. Ravenholt to denote all the diseases resulting from the use of tobacco in its various forms. He pointed out that tobaccosis is, perhaps, the deadliest plague that has affected mankind. The current estimates show over 500,000 people are dying yearly from its use. Plagues caused by microorganisms cause symptoms quickly and are easily identifiable but tobaccosis is an insidious disease with an extremely long latency period of years or decades before a symptom appears. People are reluctant to give up this addicting substance. This is a photograph of an elderly woman using snuff in the mid 1850s. It is one of the earliest images documenting tobacco use.

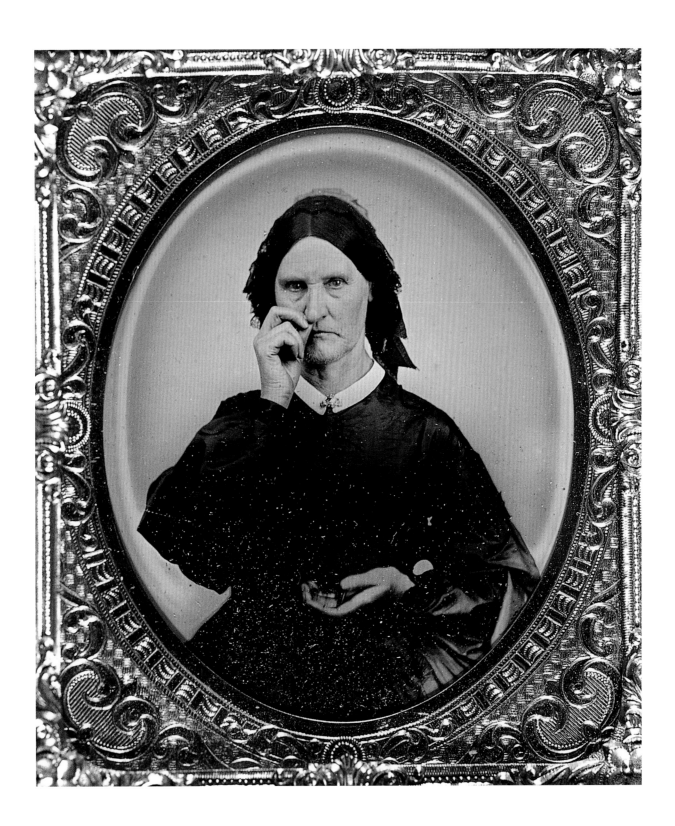

6
Dr. George Cammann:
Inventor of the Binaural Stethoscope, 'America's Instrument'

Mathew Brady, Photographer
Carte de Visite
New York
circa 1856

The stethoscope, the chest disease specialist's essential tool was practically improved by New York physician George Cammann. In 1852, Dr. Cammann perfected his binaural instrument but did not publish his results until January 1855, with a report in *The New York Medical Times*. The binaural instrument greatly intensified sound. The development of rubber tubing in the 1850s had made the construction of a binaural instrument possible. Cammann simply created a duplex portal over the stethoscope head for the rubber tubing. During the nineteenth century hundreds of modifications were made to the design to get better hearing qualities and ambient sound reduction. The earliest attempt at producing a binaural scope was in 1829 by Nicholas Comins, M.D. He was attempting to lessen the uncomfortable positions a physician had to assume to fully examine a patient with a monaural stethoscope. Other innovators who attempted to improve the binaural scope were Drs. Sheppard, Lynch, Williams, Walshe, Quain, Loomis, Alison and Clark. Some even devised a stethoscope in which each ear had its own separate headpiece so each hand could then move over the chest or back getting sounds from different areas. It was confusing and if used in that manner didn't allow localization. In 1866, New York's noted physician Austin Flint recommended use of the binaural scope over the monaural model and it soon became America's instrument. In 1885, Dr. Ford invented the bell shaped head, which improved hearing low pitched chest sounds. It became a popular and familiar headpiece. The diaphragm head allowed hearing higher pitched sounds. The bell and diaphragm headpieces were combined with a pivot screw in the twentieth century to become the familiar stethoscope of the mid-century.

The advantages of binaural over monaural designed were significant, but generated some controversy especially in Europe. In Europe the monaural stethoscope remained the essential instrument until well into the twentieth century and were produced well into the mid-twentieth century. These monographs will visually document the persistent European use of the monaural scope. Photographs will clearly show that usage as well as the practice of simply laying the head on the back or chest to hear chest sounds, in lieu of using a stethoscope. The binaural stethoscope did however become the icon of the physician in the twentieth century.

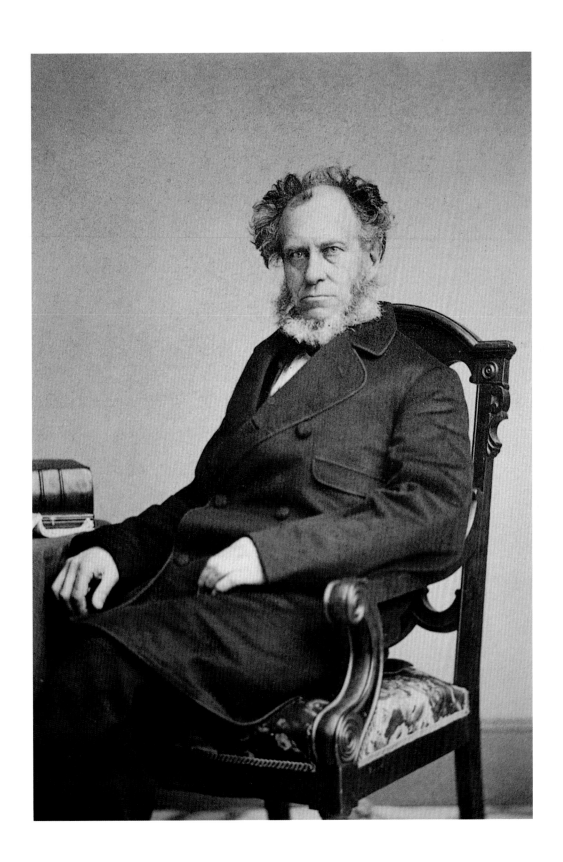

7

MEDICAL STUDENTS STUDYING

AMBROTYPE, HAND COLORED
CIRCA 1856

As photographic techniques and technology advanced posing and presentation changed. Each decade produced a fresh style of visual imagery. This photograph is typical of the 1850s. Taken as an initiation rite into medicine, students posed with the paraphernalia of their medical education. Books and body parts were the preferred props. Many of these early photographs portray several students learning together over body parts. These images predate the soon to be common photograph of students posing with their dissected cadaver. These dissection photographs had to wait until faster film was available for indoor photography. All these images are symbolic overtures to the familiar Rembrandt painting of *The Anatomy Lesson*, which was often found reproduced and hanging on the walls of medical institutions. These fledgling doctors were simply identifying themselves with medicine's oldest, best known, visual tradition.

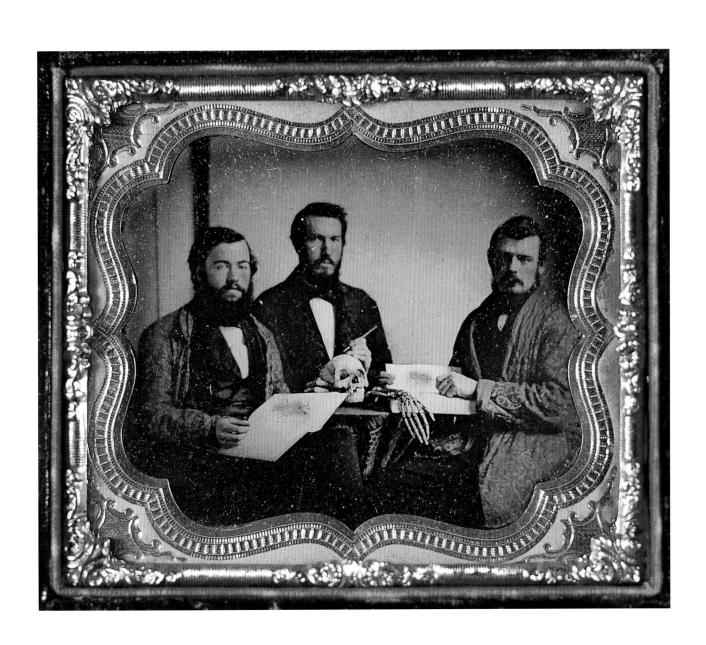

8
Blood Letting by Phlebotomy: Opening an Arm Vein
Tintype
circa 1860

Despite the fact that blood letting was common practice, photographs of nineteenth century bloodletting are very rare; only a handful are known and all are in the Burns Collection. This photograph of a frontier physician and patient illustrates the classic pose from century old tradition as depicted in engravings. The patient holds a stick to steady his arm and a bowl is suspended between the knees. The photograph was hand colored to highlight the bleeding.

For over two thousand years bloodletting was the backbone of medical practice. Western medicine adopted the Greek concept of the humoral theory of disease. Their belief was that good health depended on the proper balance of the four body humors, blood being the easiest of the humors to manipulate. Removing blood, theoretically and in practice, changed the proportion of the humors. A heroic therapy was developed by noted American physician, Dr. Benjamin Rush, where as much as 25% of the blood was removed. Bleeding in severe illnesses was done repeatedly often 30 or more ounces at a time. Traditional wisdom advised bleeding until the patient was unconscious. Children were bled until their lips turned blue. The effect of blood letting on a seriously ill, feverish, agitated or even delirious patient was immediate. They became calm, cool and pale. This treatment resulted in cardiovascular collapse, shock and often death, especially in a sick, debilitated person.

Blood letting was finally discredited with the development of medical, statistical analysis by French physicians in the mid-nineteenth century. In 1860, one astute author wrote, "If the employment of the lancet was abolished altogether, it would perhaps save annually a greater number of lives than in any one year the sword has ever destroyed."

The public was convinced of the necessity of blood letting even on healthy patients so that physicians routinely performed the procedure especially in the spring to change the body humors for the season. Blood letting was also an important part of allergy and respiratory disease treatment. The changes in antibody and blood cell production may even have had a beneficial effect. In 'lung and cardiac congestion' it actually helps and remains an integral part of medical management for pulmonary edema, blood dyscrasias, polycythemia vera and cardiac congestion. Every modern patient knows the current form of blood letting. The drawing of blood for lab tests is one of the most important procedures in evaluating a patient.

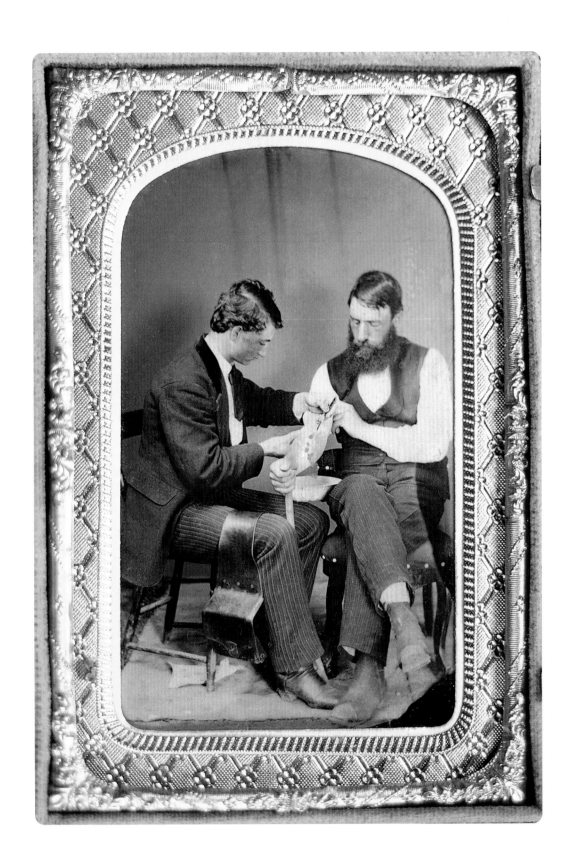

9
Homeopathic Physician with His Vials of Medicine
Ambrotype
circa 1858

Homeopathic physicians followed the philosophy of Christian F.S. Hahnemann, M.D. (1755-1843), using extremely diluted medications. They routinely posed for photographs displaying their small medicinal vials. In this image the doctor is pouring medication. Unlike traditional doctors, homeopaths did not interfere with the natural course of disease, many of which were self-limiting. On the other hand mainstream 'allopathic' physicians used powerful, often poisonous, remedies in doses that often caused more harm than good. In the first half of the nineteenth century the main treatment modality was the aggressive treatment known as 'heroic therapy'. Devised by noted Philadelphia physician, Benjamin Rush (1745-1813), a signer of the Declaration of Independence, this therapeutic practice may have killed as many patients as it helped. Heroic therapy subjected the patients to repeated bleeding, purging, vomiting and blistering. Respiratory diseases such as pneumonia, asthma, catarrh and diphtheria, were treated by this regime. It's no wonder the public responded to the less aggressive therapies offered by herbalists, homeopaths and the many other sects offering minimally invasive therapies. The motto for homeopathy was - Simila Similibus Curantur - or 'Like Cures Like'. In practice, infinitesimally small doses of a medication were given, diluted to absurd extremes so in effect the patient was receiving no medication at all. As strange as this may sound, it was a great deal safer than the heroic therapy. The germ theory of disease and other notable medical advancements relating to the cause of disease lead homeopaths to gradually embrace traditional medicine and by the mid-twentieth century they had been drawn into the mainstream of medical practices.

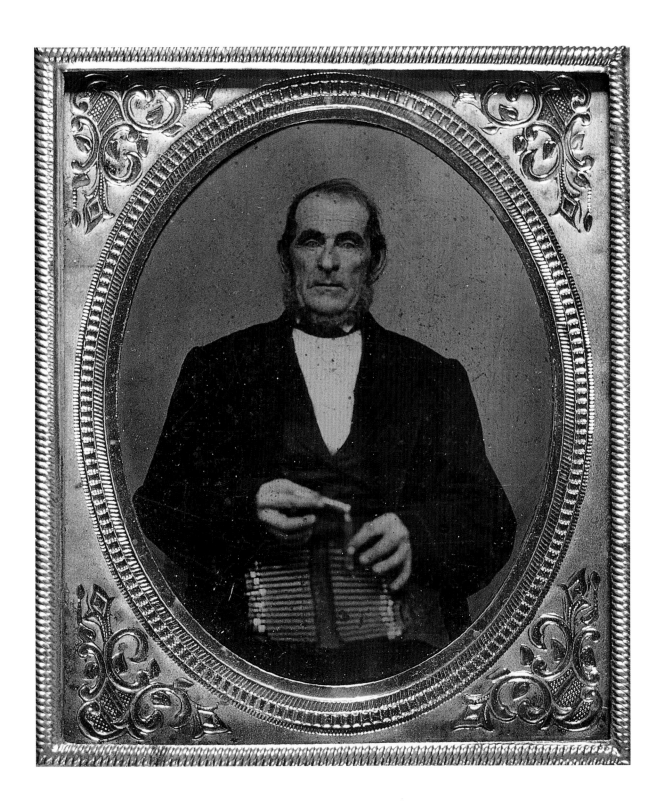

TRACHEOTOMY: ANCIENT TECHNIQUE FOR ACUTE RESPIRATORY DISTRESS

ALBUMEN PRINT, 5 BY 6 INCHES
CIRCA 1859-60

This dramatic close up of a tracheotomy is the earliest photograph of the procedure. The postmortem image was taken to show the technique of using a ring with stress sutures to hold the lumen open. This infant suffered severe burns on the arms and legs and was treated with a special parchment type wound dressing. Infection and fluid loss are the main complications of burns. In this pre-antiseptic era, there were no specific attempts to combat either occurrence. However, this innovative dressing may have been a pioneering attempt to cover skin. Respiratory distress was also a recognized complication of several maladies and the tracheotomy has been a known surgical intervention since ancient times. By the seventeenth century to assist breathing in wounds and cases of foreign bodies in the larynx, trocars and cannulas were being used by a few surgeons who inserted them into the trachea. Although it was Thomas Feinus in 1649 who first used the word tracheotomy, it was Lorenz Heister who introduced the term into general usage in his 1750s text, *A General System of Surgery*. Laryngotomy and bronchotomy were terms defined in the nineteenth century and used together with tracheotomy. Armond Trousseau, M.D. (1801-1867), promoted both the procedure and the term tracheotomy. Nineteenth century physicians attempted to access the success of the procedure. In 1884, Viennese physician, Alois Monti (1839-1909), collected 12,736 cases of laryngeal diphtheria treated with tracheotomy, the mortality rate was 73.4%. While this sounds high, prior to this practice the mortality rate was about 100%. Tracheotomies for laryngeal diphtheria became firmly established by the mid-nineteenth century but with the introduction of immunization for diphtheria there was a dramatic decrease in the use of the procedure. Other conditions treated in the nineteenth century by tracheotomy included epilepsy, tuberculosis, tetanus, and various surgical procedures. This photograph provides evidence it was also used in burn cases. An English surgeon named Chovell attempted to use the tracheotomy in an innovative money making scheme. In the 1780s with the payment of a substantial fee Chovell persuaded a condemned prisoner he could save his life if allowed to perform a tracheotomy the night before he was to be hanged. The operation was deemed successful but the 'patient' died a few minutes after he was cut down. The doctor blamed his failure on the man's excessive weight. He was, however, a hero among the criminal class for his clever ploy.

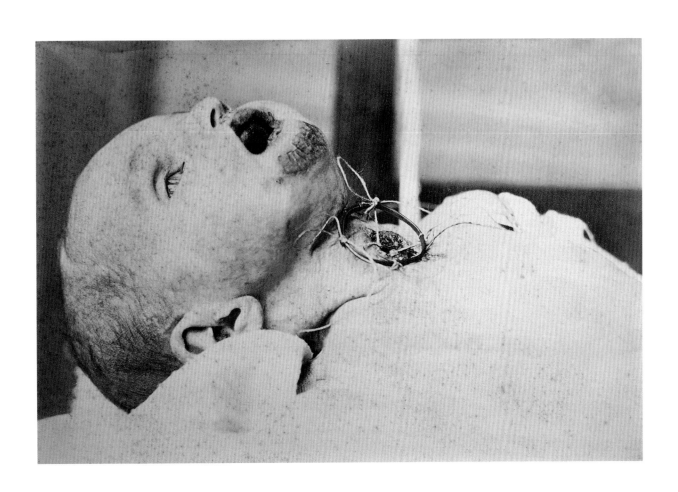

11
The Otoscope: A Specialty is Born
Ambrotype
circa 1860

This 1860s English ambrotype is the earliest known photograph of an ear examination. In photography's earliest era, of all nations English practitioners seem to have favored posing with new instruments. This doctor is using an early otoscope to examine the child's ear. Ear and mastoid infections were so common that they were believed to be a normal part of childhood. The mid-nineteenth century saw the invention of several diagnostic tools for the head and neck. With these specialized tools medical specialties were born. Ophthalmology was established with the invention of the ophthalmoscope in 1851 by Hermann von Helmhotz, M.D. (1821-1894). Within a few years the upper respiratory tract disease specialty of otorhinolaryngology was founded with the invention of two specialized instruments. These were the laryngoscope, invented by voice teacher Manuel Garcia (1805-1906) in 1855 and the otoscope, invented by Anton von Tröltsch (1829-1890) in 1860. The promotion and practical application of laryngoscopy by Ludwig Turck, M.D. (1810-1868) and Johann Czermack, M.D. (1828-1873) firmly established the field. Austrian otolaryngologists soon became the world's leaders in this specialty. Physicians seemed to adapt to new instrumentation more quickly than new concepts of disease care, such as antiseptic and asepsis. It should also be noted that with the birth of new specialties minorities and women were more easily allowed to enter these fields of practice as master surgeons and physicians in the hierarchy had little interest in them. The sub-specialty field of otoscopy was championed by the Viennese physician Adam Politzer, M.D. (1835-1920), the Austrian physician who invented head mirror. Aside from his numerous discoveries related to ear disease and its treatment, in 1865, he became the first person to successfully photograph the tympanic membrane. His photographs were later used in his famous 1896 publication, *Atlas der Beleutungbilder des Trommelfels*. Dr. Politzer is considered the father of modern, scientific otology. His clinic served between 15-20,000 patients a year. During his 46 years of teaching he received over 7,000 foreign physicians. Politzer's influence reached well into the twentieth century.

Ear infections were among the most frequent complications of upper respiratory tract disease and often cause of deafness. Syphilis, tuberculosis and other common ear infections caused not only chronic drainage but mastoiditis. The main therapeutic modalities at this time were surgical drainage and local antiseptic treatment. During the nineteenth century ear disease and its treatment played a key role in the cause and management of respiratory tract infections. As children were especially prone to these infections treatment fell into the domain of the general practitioner. The sheer number of cases and severe complications served as an impetus for establishment of the specialized otologist. With the advent of antibiotics and decline in infectious ear disease the otologist's concern turned toward restoration of hearing.

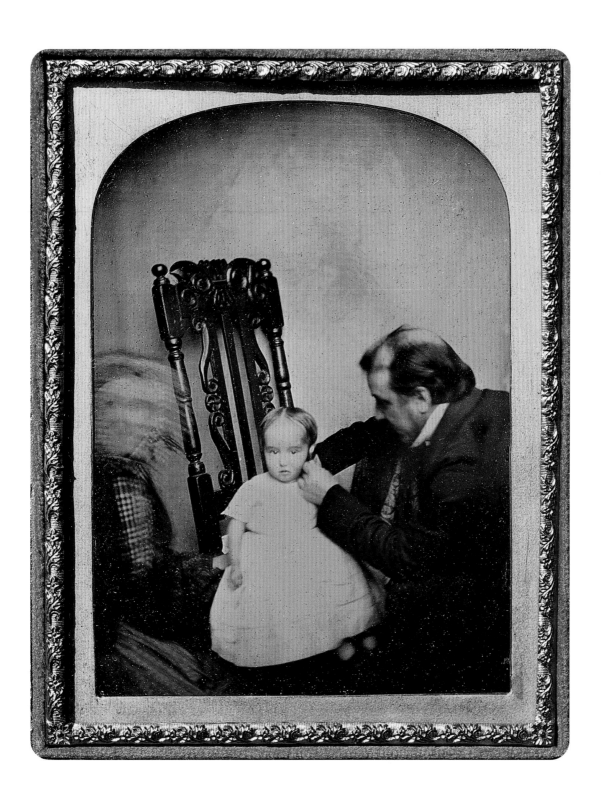

12
Army Surgeon, Dr. S. Baird Wolf, About to Amputate an Arm

Carte de Visite
Paducah, Kentucky
1864

Maintenance of airway ventilation and respiratory control was, and still is, one of the most important concerns during surgery. Some surgeons during the Civil War era decided that having the patient sit upright was a more natural position for some major operations. There are only approximately a dozen photographs taken during the Civil War that depict actual battlefield hospital surgery in progress. Two of these images show the patient being operated upon while sitting up. In the pre-anesthetic era surgeons were rated by how fast they could remove a limb. A master surgeon could perform an arm amputation in about a minute and a leg amputation in under three minutes. This speed was deemed quick enough to avoid any respiratory problems and allow the anesthetized patient to sit upright. During the war many physicians joined the military to learn how to operate as there was a seemingly endless supply of wounded. However, it seems to be a safe assumption that Dr. Wolf was a master surgeon before the war as he was not only skilled enough to perform the procedure with the patient in this position but also have the surgery visually documented.

This photograph is probably a studio posed view and most likely taken to show the position and operative preparation. Except for a bowl to catch blood and tissue, the procedure is in the classic form of the era and offers a wealth of information on the operating standards. The lack of sterile technique is obvious. Surgeons and assistants operated in their ordinary clothes and the patient still wore his uniform. The only special garb of the era was, perhaps, an apron used by the surgeon. The apron enabled him to wipe the blood and debris from his knife and bone saw. Most surgeons used the same apron and unwashed linen from case to case whether the patient had been infected or not. The discovery of anesthesia offered the patient freedom from pain and granted the surgeon extended time to operate. However, extensive procedures were often to the detriment of the patient as mortality was still extremely high due to infection. The practice of antiseptic operating and the germ theory of disease were post war discoveries. Viewed in that light, it was certainly understandable that post-operative infections with their laudable pus were considered normal.

The glazed look on this patient's face indicates he may be under the effects of an anesthetic. A bottle of ether or, perhaps, chloroform, is held under his nose. Double tourniquets delineate the amputation site. The position of surgeon, assistant and anesthetist is standard. On the back of this photograph is documentation of the case with the photographers printed logo, 'D.P. Barr, Army Photographer, Paducah, Ky.' This is an unusual war time signature as most war photographers were in the field and did not have studios. Apparently Barr, based with an army group, had a studio on the post. Dr. Baird took this opportunity to have a photograph taken for use as a teaching tool for surgeons inexperienced with the treatment of war wounds.

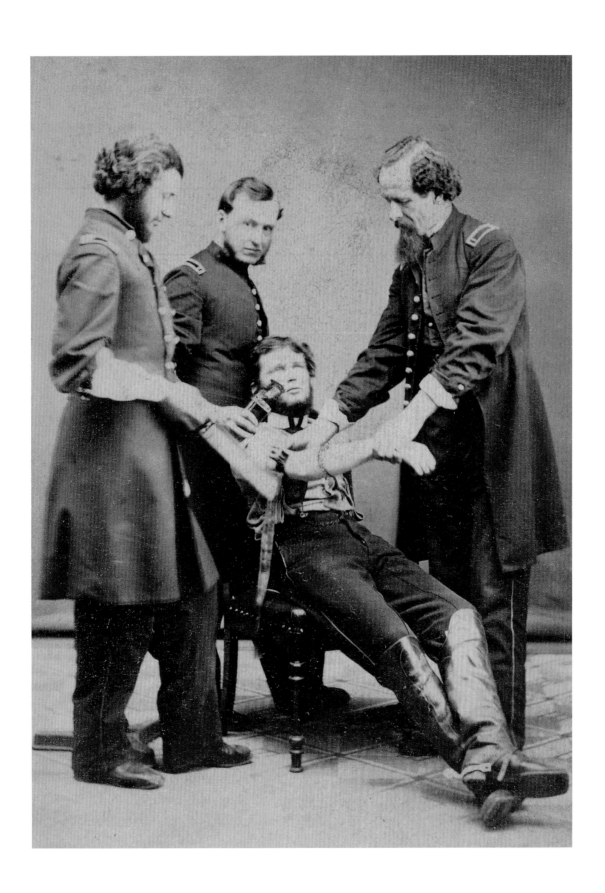

Erysepilas: An Abnormal Wound Infection in the Civil War

Private John B. Shadle, Co. C, 87th Pennsylvania Volunteers
Harewood US Army General Hospital, Washington DC
Reed Brockway Bontecou, M.D., Surgeon in Charge
Carte de Visite
April 1865

In the pre-antiseptic era, it was 'normal' for patients with open wounds to contract an infection with 'laudable pus'. However, the following five conditions were readily identifiable as abnormal infections: tetanus and osteomyelitis, and a trio of highly contagious states - pyemia (septicemia), erysepilas and hospital gangrene. Any of these last three were the cause of the dreaded infection 'hospitalism', a secondary infection usually contracted during the long hospital stays common in the Civil War era. Pyemia, the deadliest of these infections, had a mortality rate of 97%. Approximately 20% of wounded soldiers had these secondary infections.

Private Shadle had been wounded at the Battle of Petersburg, Virginia on April 2, 1865, seven days before the end of the Civil War. He suffered a gunshot wound to his right thumb, which was amputated at a field hospital. Ten days later he was admitted to Harewood US Army General Hospital, Washington, DC where he soon contracted erysepilas. Despite the obvious toxicity of his disease, Shadle managed to calmly sit for this formal hospital photograph taken by Reed B. Bontecou, M.D., Surgeon in Charge of the hospital. Shadle was treated with "repeated deep and free incisions, which drained the entire arm" together with "liberal external use of tincture of ferric chloride." He was one of the lucky few who survived erysepilas. He was discharged June 1, 1865 just two months after his wounding.

Methods of combating erysepilas were often more extreme. For example, Confederate General, William Hugh Young, after receiving severe shrapnel wounds of the left leg, was belatedly taken to a field hospital. By that time, his leg had developed both erysepilas and gangrene. Young was immediately strapped to a stretcher and without anesthetic, watched, as his leg was drenched with nitric acid. The acid did its antiseptic work with sickening efficiency. His life was spared but his leg was grotesquely scarred. Nitric acid was routinely used by Federal physicians, as it was an effective way of dealing with hospitalism in extremity wounds. Chest, head and abdominal wounds, however, could not be treated with any of the caustic chemical measures and secondary infections were usually fatal. Southern physicians while also using nitric acid would sometimes apply maggots to the wound. This was a safe and effective method for the removal of dead tissue.

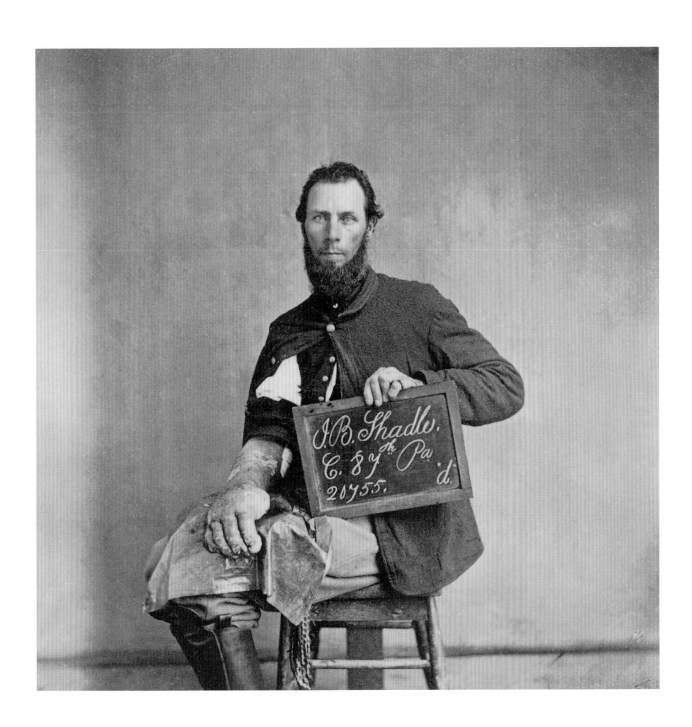

14
CHEST WOUNDS IN THE CIVIL WAR

HAREWOOD USA GENERAL HOSPITAL, WASHINGTON DC
REED BROCKWAY BONTECOU, M.D., SURGEON IN CHARGE
ALBUMEN PRINT, 4 BY 6 INCHES
1865

Presented for the first time is a photographic compilation of Civil War soldiers with various gun shot wounds of the chest. These cases and histories are from the original albums of Harewood Hospital's Chief Surgeon, Reed Brockway Bontecou, M.D. Dr. Bontecou was the most prolific of all medical photographers and the largest contributor to the Army Medical Museum's collection during the war. These photographs represent the first pioneer effort to visually document and teach surgeons about chest wounds.

War is usually responsible for medical progress as the large number of cases make it possible to test and compare various therapies. During the Civil War several areas of medicine advanced. Standards of physician competence and education were established. Treatment of penetrating chest wounds and techniques in plastic surgery of the head and neck were improved. A hospital for neurological wounds was founded in Philadelphia at Turners Lane. Six enormous volumes were published, titled, *The Medical and Surgical History of the War of the Rebellion.* They not only set a standard for statistical analysis of medical care but also included evaluation of treatment and presented interesting case reports. The hermetically sealing of penetrating chest wounds has saved thousands of lives since that time. On June 25, 1863, US Army Assistant Surgeon, Benjamin Howard, addressed a letter to Surgeon General Alexander Hammond describing his new mode of treatment.

> After cleaning the wound, and removing foreign bodies; bring the opposite edges together, and retain them in accurate apposition by metallic sutures; carefully dry the wound...pour a few drops of collodion so as to saturate it. (the dressing cloth); let it dry; then apply one or two additional coats of collodion and repeat the process until satisfied that the wound is hermetically sealed. A dose of lint may then be applied.

Howard then pointed out that the lung was able to re-absorb trapped fluid and air and then re-expand. One of his most important observations documented was that, "The most distressing symptom, dyspnea is relieved immediately." In Europe Howard's therapy was sarcastically nicknamed 'The American Plan.' As Europe was the world's medical leader few innovations developed in America were given much credence. Only the discovery of general anesthesia was accepted quickly. However, Dr. Howard's innovation of hermetically sealing chest wounds gradually became the world standard.

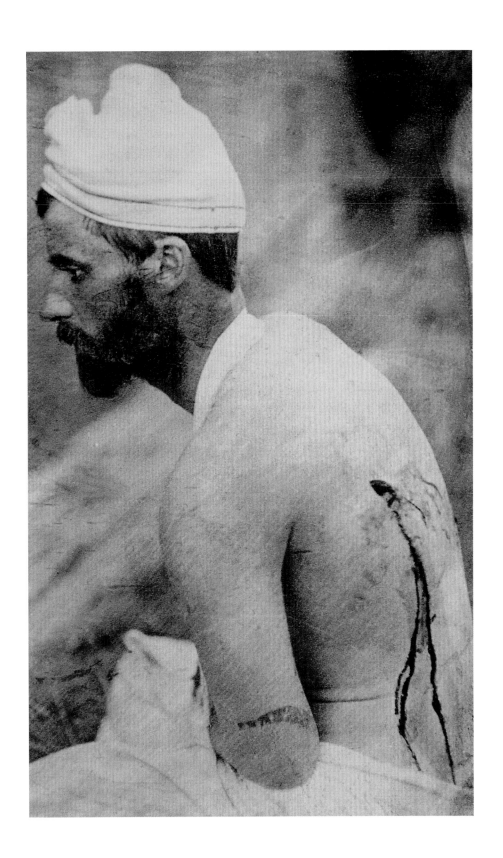

Gunshot Wound of the Chest: A Civil War Teaching Case

Abner C. Emery, Shot in the Chest, 2nd Lt. Co. X, 2nd Maine Cavalry
US Army Medical Museum
Carte de Visite
1863

The surgeon drew the suspected path of the bullet on this photograph. By putting together a collection of 'wound' photographs documented with their treatment and survival rates, surgeons were able to teach and improve both techniques and medical care during the Civil War. This photograph is from the original Army Medical Museum collection established during the war. The original set of photographs taken by Dr. Bontecou and presented on the following pages was reproduced in the size of a calling card, known as a carte de visite. They form a portion of the museum's 'contributed' photograph collection. The written legend, "Contr Photo 62", is the identification assigned the card. About 1000 of these cards were dispersed by museum personnel in the early part of the twentieth century.

US Army Surgeon General, William Alexander Hammond, M.D. (1828-1900), conceived and planned the creation of the medical museum in Washington, DC. His idea was to provide pathological specimens of war wounds and diseases for study in order to improve the care of the sick and wounded. In Circular No. 2, May 21, 1862, Hammond laid down the principles for the museum. The Army Medical Museum evolved into the Armed Forces Institute of Pathology, which ultimately was responsible for numerous advances in medicine.

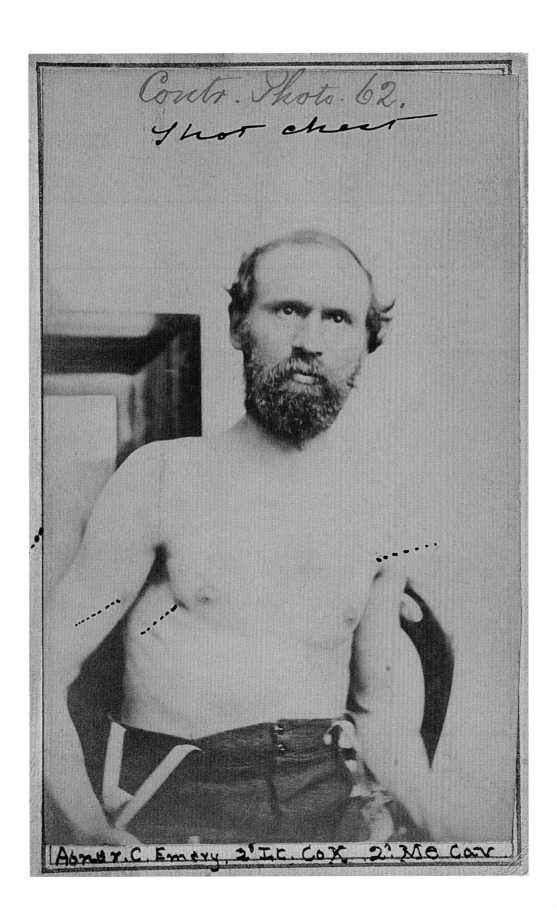

Contr. Shots. 62,
Shot chest

Abner C. Emery 2'Lt. Co K. 2' Mo Cav

16
Gunshot Wound of the Chest with Pyemia

Edward Morgan, Private, Co. C 15th New York Cavalry
Harewood US Army General Hospital, Washington DC
Reed Brockway Bontecou, M.D., Surgeon in Charge
Albumen Print, 4 by 6 inches
April 1865

This photograph was chosen from a special album Dr. Bontecou created for use as a teaching aid in his own hospital. He also included photographs taken by other surgeons of interesting cases. These 4 by 6 inch photographs were the largest sized print made during the war. Dr. Bontecou outlined in red the path of the bullet and also in this case colored in some 'blood.' Private Morgan lived about three weeks after his wound was infected. The case history reads as follows:

Edward Morgan, private Co. C, 15th New York Cav., aged 22, was admitted to Harewood Hospital April 5, 1865, suffering from a gunshot wound left side, ball entering below scapula exit near spine in dorsal region, perforating pleural cavity, fracturing two ribs. Wounded Apr. 1st, at Battle of South-Side Railroad. On admission the constitution state of patient was very good, apparently suffering but little from his wound. The extent of injury could not be ascertained; the parts in very good condition. The patient did tolerable well up to April 28, when pyemic symptoms appeared, from that period he steadily sank and died May 1st 1865. Treatment: Alternatives and supporting throughout. On post mortem examination found the ninth and tenth ribs, left side severely fractured and the pleural cavity perforated. A quantity of serum slightly mixed with pus was found in left pleural cavity; abscesses were found on surface of lower lobe left lung; right lung appeared to be normal; no pus was found in the auxiliary or femoral veins; heart normal; liver and spleen also in good condition.

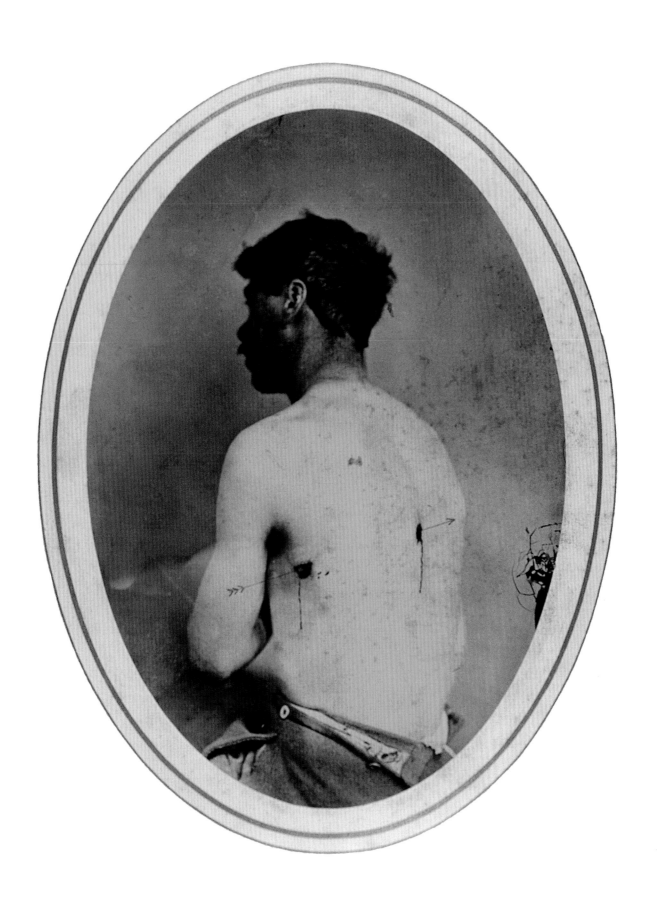

17

SURVIVAL OF GUN SHOT WOUND OF THE CHEST WITH ERYSEPILAS

DANIEL RICH, CO. B, 55TH PENNSYLVANIA VOLUNTEERS
BEAUFORT, SOUTH CAROLINA
REED BROCKWAY BONTECOU, M.D., SURGEON IN CHARGE
ALBUMEN PRINT, 4 BY 6 INCHES
1862

Dr. Bontecou recorded this case early in the war when he was in charge of a military hospital in Beaufort, South Carolina. The survival of a patient with erysepilas from a gun shot wound of the lung is extraordinarily rare. The typical severity of erysepilas is shown in photograph number 13. The following is a direct quote from Dr. Bontecou:

Daniel Rich, Co. B, 55th Pennsylvania vols., aged 21 years, wounded at the battle of Pocotoligo, Oct. 22nd and admitted to Hospital no. 1, Beaufort, S.C., Oct. 24th, 1862, with gunshot wound of the chest, the ball entering at the sterno-clavicular articulation of the right side, and emerging five inches distance between first and second ribs of the left side, penetrating the sternum in its course. He spit blood in small quantities at the moment of injury, but walked to the placed of embarkation, a distance of five or six miles. He was obliged to lie on his back, and had lost power in both arms to some extent. When admitted here, his face was flushed and dusky, coarse rhales were audible in his bronchia, and accelerated pulse, evidently some inflammatory mischief going on in the lungs or bronchia. I did not deem it advisable to bleed, as his wound, he said, had bled much ever since his injury.
 Oct. 25th. Excitement of vascular system less, the medicine had sickened him and acted on the bowels. His spine seems perfectly rigid and the cervical vertebrae are tender to the touch.
  Oct. 27th. Respiration easy; wound suppurating. Until 31st inst., when the soft parts covering the upper part of the sternum had become red and fluctuated. The discharge could, with some difficulty, be forced out of the wound in the left side. I therefore made a free incision in this, and gave the discharge vent. An opening into the chest through the sternum was apparent to the finger introduced through the wound. The new wound, as well as the others, discharges freely, good pus, and 4th, but the stiffness of spine and inability to move the arms remain.
  Nov. 18th. He can now move his arms somewhat, and sits up an hour. Cough disappeared. I think it was when he first sat up, and thus allowed the matter to run out that this symptom disappeared.
  Dec. 1st. Rich has been walking around the ward. He walks as if all the parts above the pelvis were ossified together. Yesterday a small piece of bone came out of the opening over the sternum, and was of the size of a ten cent piece.
  Dec. 20th. Rich has been doing very well. Erysipelas has successively invaded chest, left arm, shoulder and back, but is now disappearing. Very little discharge from the wounds.
  Dec. 28th. Sent to northern hospital, per steamer - Star of the South.

 Despite the serious nature of chest wounds some did survive not only the initial wound, but the secondary infection. This lucky soldier not only survived he continued to serve after his miraculous recover from erysepilas of the chest and upper body. Dr. Bontecou adds in his own hand "He was subsequently put in the Invalid Corps and served in the ranks until the close of the war. (signed) RBB."

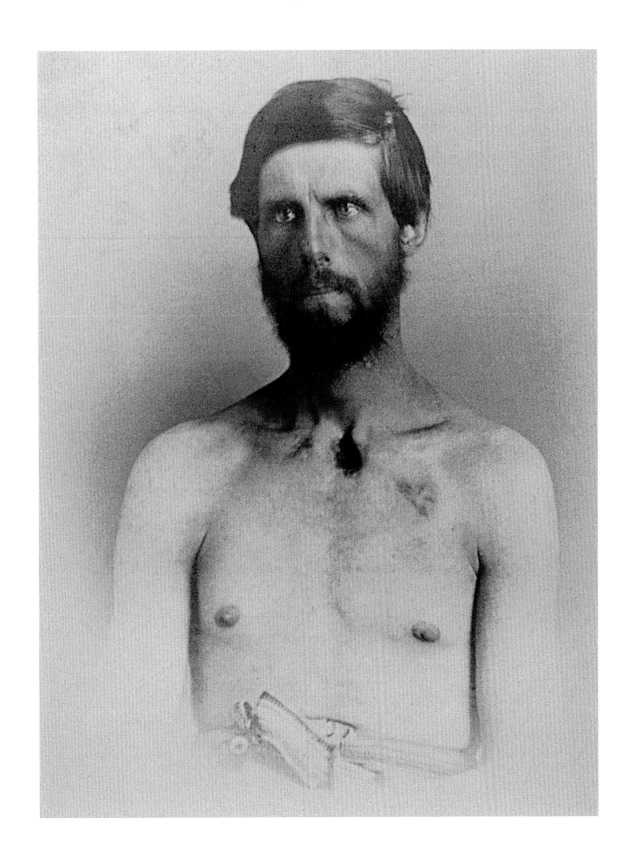

Paracentesis of the Thorax for 'Traumatic' Pleurisy, GSW Chest

Israel Spotts, Corporal Co. G, 200th Pa. Volunteers
Harewood US Army General Hospital, Washington DC
Reed Brockway Bontecou, M.D., Surgeon in Charge
Albumen Print, 4 by 6 inches
March 1865

This patient sits showing his pulmonary drainage tube and collection pan. Dr. Bontecou's note suggests he had cured this patient. Other records proved the seriousness of the pulmonary infection.

Corporal Israel Spotts, Co. G, 200th Pa. Vols., aged 24, was admitted to Harewood U.S.A., General Hospital, April 5th, 1865, suffering from gunshot wound of the back, dorsal region, ball entered the chest opposite the fourth dorsal vertebrae, between the spine and scapula. Wounded, March 25th, 1865, at the battle of Petersburgh, Va.. On admission, the condition of injured parts and constitutional state of patient were good; did very well for awhile, wound healing kindly, but towards the early part of the month of May the chest became enormously distended with effusion, harassing cough, anxiety of countenance, oppressed breathing and symptoms of empyema. An operation being necessary to relieve the patient parenthesis thoracis was performed by Surgeon R. B. Bontecou, U.S. Vols., May 9th, 1865, by freely opening the chest at right posterior and lateral aspect, between eighth and ninth ribs and about six pints of sanious pus removed, no anesthetic used; the patient felt at once relieved, did remarkably well after the operation; was doing well and in tolerably good condition when he deserted from this hospital, May 28th, 1865. Treatment in this case was simple dressings, anodynes and supporting throughout.

Dr. Bontecou's photograph album ends with the story of Corporal Spotts, his survival and with his 'dissertion' (from the hospital). One of the achievements of the war was publication of the statistical analysis of all cases of disease, wounds and injuries over a 15 year period. In the *Medical And Surgical History of the War of the Rebellion, Surgical Volume 2, Part 1* which documents chest wounds, Corporal Spotts' story continues with a slightly different ending. He was furloughed and sent to his home at Hammondstown, Pennsylvania. Dr. Stichley, attending physician states:

Saw soldier after he reached home; found him suffering from empyema. After he was home a few days an operation was performed on him, removing two or three quarts of pus from his chest. Operation had to be performed every two or three weeks. The bullet was still in the lung. He lived in this condition for about two months. Death resulted September 20th, 1865 from exhaustion produced by suppuration.

Corporal Spotts' case was an example in which "paracentesis of the thorax was performed, (for) traumatic pleurisy, with effusion, following gunshot wound that apparently did not penetrate the pleural cavity. This photograph is considered one of the most artistic Civil War medical photographs. A copy of the image is in the collection of New York's Metropolitan Museum of Art.

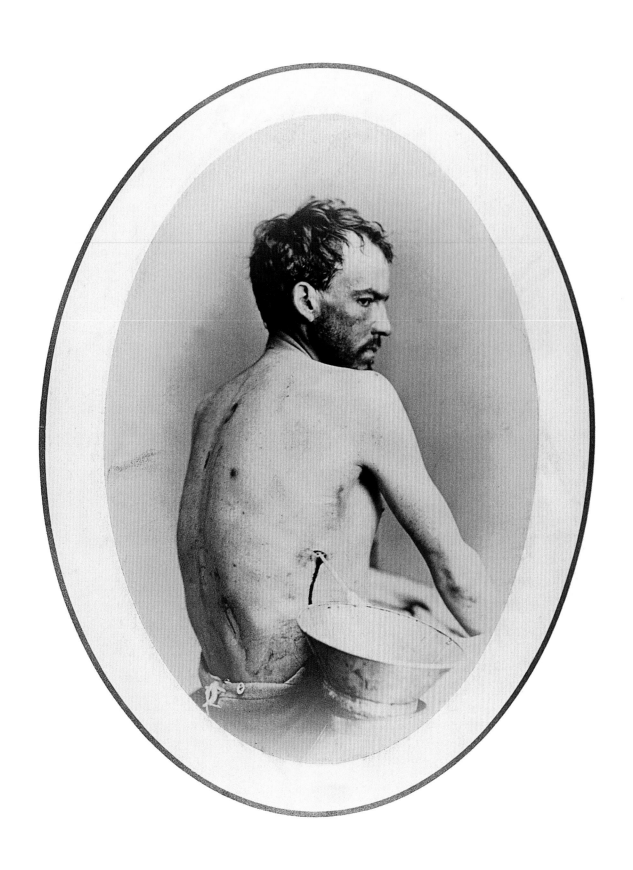

FATAL GUN SHOT WOUND OF CHEST, 'PARACENTESIS & THORACASIS'

MEDEAD BECK, PRIVATE, CO. G. 11TH VERMONT VOLUNTEERS
HAREWOOD US ARMY GENERAL HOSPITAL, WASHINGTON DC
REED BROCKWAY BONTECOU, M.D., SURGEON IN CHARGE
ALBUMEN PRINT 4 BY 6 INCHES
APRIL 1865

Infected chest wounds were usually fatal as the previous case illustrates. This case is an example of the frustration felt when treating these cases in the pre-antiseptic/asepsis era.

Medead Beck, private, Co G. 11th Vt. Vols. Aged 46 was admitted Harewood USA General Hospital April 12 1865 suffering from gunshot of thorax left side, ball entering at fourth rib about two inches from sternum perforating right lung and passing out just below inferior angle of scapular. Wounded, April 2nd 1865 at the battle of Petersburgh Va. On admission, the injured parts were intolerably good condition, the patient however suffering from dyspnae, extensive emphesyema of surrounding cellular tissues, anxious expression of countenance and symptoms of pneumothorax; Chest freely opened by posterior incision and a large amount of sanious pus removed. Result unfavorable. Treat: Supporting. Patient died, April 17th 1865, from exhaustion. On postmortem examined the fourth rib fractured anteriorly and eighth and ninth ribs posteriorly; right lung perforated.

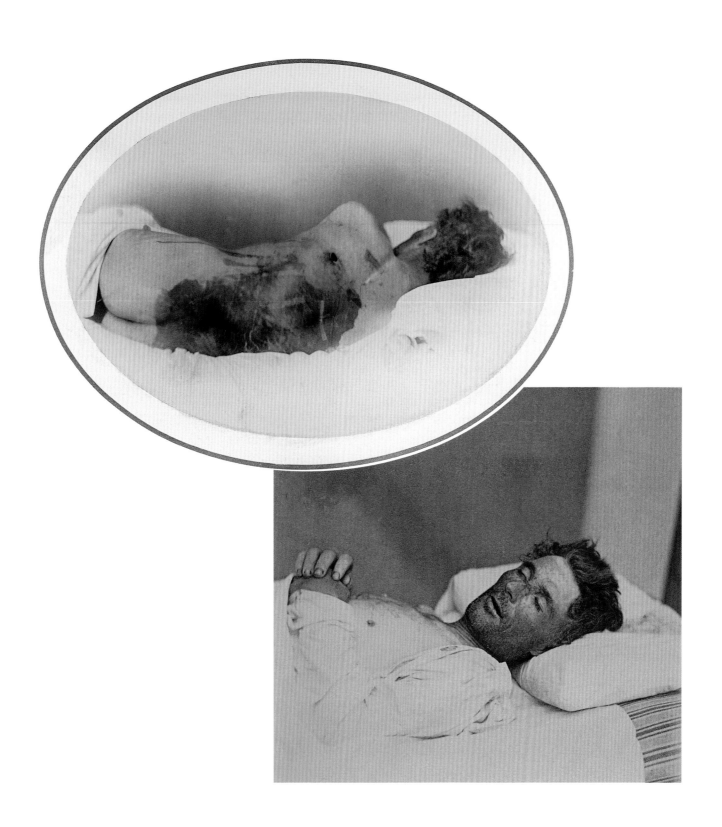

20
Gunshot Wound of the Chest, Emerging Below Sternum

Frederick A. Bentley, Private, Co. A. 185th New York Volunteers
Harewood US Army General Hospital, Washington DC
Reed Brockway Bontecou, M.D., Surgeon in Charge
Albumen Print, 4 by 6 inches
April 1865

One of the fascinating aspects of gunshot wounds in the Civil War was the sheer luck involved in survival. As all wounds became infected, the secondary infection incurred, frequently with long hospital stays, playing a key role in survival. Similar wounds, even when superficial, offered a wide range of outcomes. This patient spent almost two months at the hospital and had an uneventful recovery.

Frederick A. Bentley, Private, Co. A. 185th N.Y. Vols.; aged 18, native of New York, was admitted to this hospital April 2nd, 1865, with gunshot wound of side, the ball entering the left side and emerging near the medial line, below the sternum. Wounded at Stone Creek March 29th, 1865. He recovered under simple dressing, with very little stimulants, and no special diet. Transferred May 29th, 1865, to Phila.

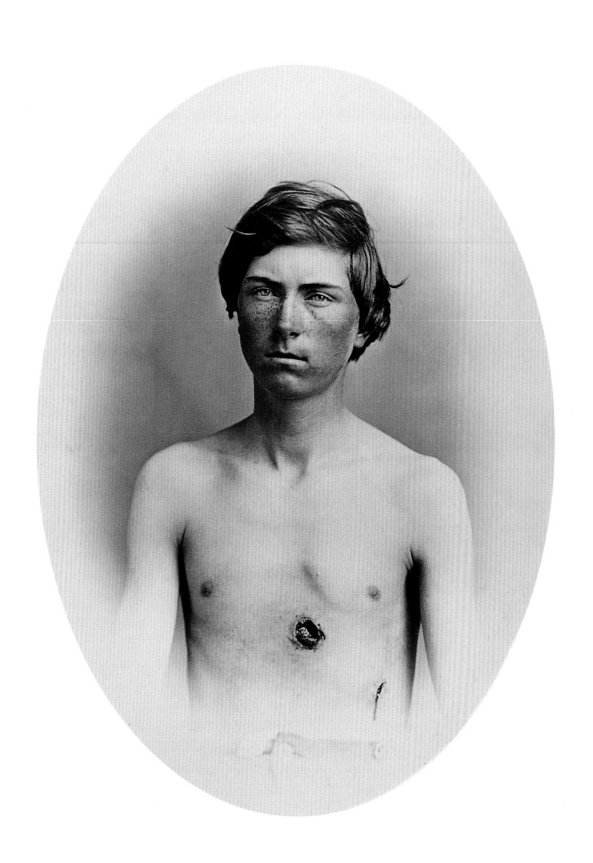

MASTECTOMY: HEALED USING EARTH DRESSING

WOODBURYTYPE, 4 BY 3 1/2 INCHES
PHILADELPHIA
1869

During the Civil War Louis Pasteur's (1822-1895) research conclusions stating putrefaction and bacteria caused fermentation were published. English surgeon, Joseph Lister (1827-1912), put Pasteur's idea into a landmark medical proposal. Since foreign matter, bacteria, dirt, etc. were the culprits in wound healing he recognized that by keeping a wound clean it would heal without infection. Lister's antiseptic wound treatment and surgical antiseptic procedures were the second greatest medical innovation of the nineteenth century (1867). With the knowledge of the fatality rate from secondary infections during the Civil War and in the light of both Pasteur's and Lister's work, physicians were certainly not responsive to the therapy suggestions of Philadelphia surgeon, Adinell Hewson, M.D. (1828-1889). He proposed an innovative operative wound treatment, using earth as the dressing.

A fascinating aspect of medical discovery is the fact that, occasionally, great ideas and advances lay hidden in old books and journals. However, open minds and new technologies are sometimes necessary to understand and implement the discoveries of the past. In 1872, Dr. Addinell Hewson published, *Earth as a Topical Application in Surgery*. He describes his treatment of wounds and operative cases by the application of earth to the wound and the accompanying acceleration of the healing process. He details ninety-three cases including ulcers, burns, gunshot wounds and operations such as this mastectomy. All wounds were dressed with his special dirt and all healed quickly, most within fifteen days. Hewson attributed this healing to the action of ozone, deoxygenation and released ammonia. It was more likely infection was inhibited by the presence of a naturally occurring antibacterial agent in the soil such as bacitracin. Unfortunately for Hewson, his work appeared at the same time Lister's antiseptic surgical technique was being promoted and widely accepted by surgeons. Packing wounds with dirt made no sense to a profession recently convinced of the necessity for cleanliness. If Hewson's findings been taken more seriously and evaluated, the age of antibiotics might have dawned a half-century sooner.

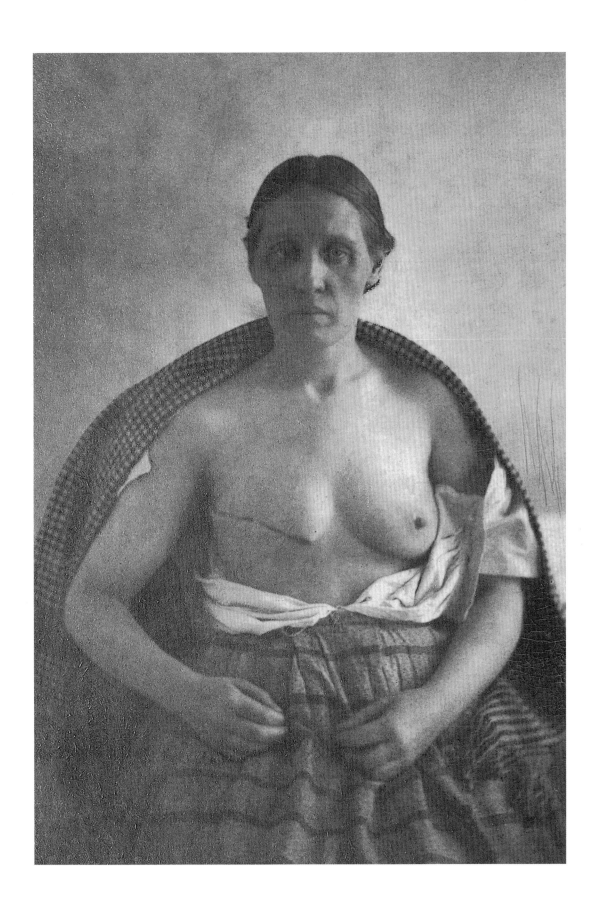

22

TUBERCULOSIS OF THE NOSE, OZENA

ALBUMEN PRINT, 4 BY 5 INCHES
CIRCA 1870

Nasal ulcers when first presented were a diagnostic problem especially early in the nineteenth century. However, as the disease progressed and the symptoms increased the diagnosis became easier. Major consideration was always given to cancer, tuberculosis or syphilis. Syphilis eroded all the tissues including bone and tuberculosis destroyed soft tissue and cartilage though the bone was left intact. Loss of the nose was a social stigma for centuries and plastic surgeons from the Renaissance onward attempted to develop procedures to improve patient appearance. Most of the inflicted used a nasal prosthesis. Men usually attached a mustache to the prosthesis, which could hide more defects. There was one problem with extensive loss of the nose that was difficult to hide, the dreaded infection 'ozena.' Ozena was an ailment of much prominence in the pre-bacteriological/antibiotic era because it accompanied many infectious and neoplastic diseases of the nose. Ozena is derived from the Greek word meaning 'to stink'. The infection of the nasal cavities resulted in a foul nasal discharge and a fetid breath. In his 1881 text, *A Manual of Diseases of the Nose and Throat*, Dr. Frank Bosworth noted that the ozena that accompanied syphilis was particularly offensive. He stated that the 'breath is often so penetrating and nauseating as to render the near presence of the sufferer not only unpleasant but almost unendurable.' Nasal douching, carbolic acid and other astringents were offered as remedies. Nasal sprays or the inhalation of various chemical vapors were often prescribed. With the development of bacteriology the organisms causing ozena were identified as *Klebsiella ozena* and *Bacillus foetidus*. With the conquest by antibiotics of tuberculosis and syphilis ozena is mainly seen today as a manifestation of atrophic rhinitis, a marked degeneration of the nasal mucosa. This occurs most commonly as a hereditary malady but is also associated with the injudicious use of nasal sprays and drops.

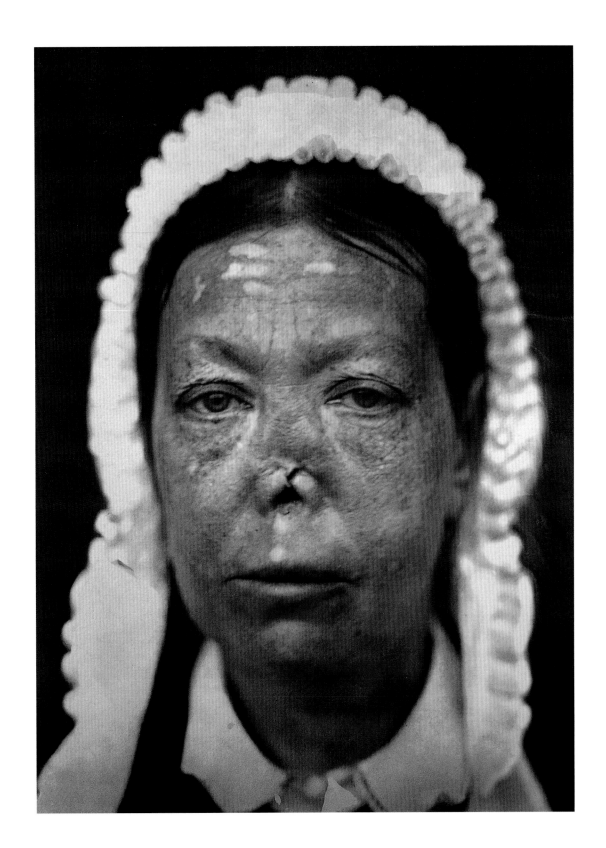

23
Scrufulide Tuberculeuse: Loss of the Nose (Lupus)
A. Montmeja, M.D.
Albumen Print, Hand Colored, 4 by 5 inches
Paris
1868

In the nineteenth century, severe upper respiratory tract disease as a complication from tuberculosis was common. The destruction and necrosis of nasal and facial tissue served as a breeding ground for other pathogens. These secondary organisms lead to ear, sinus and nasal infection. Dermatological texts often document skin manifestations of primary lung and other respiratory tract disease. Astute physicians could often diagnose a primary respiratory tract condition from the skin manifestation.

This image was published in the 1868 edition of the dermatological atlas, *Clinique Photographique de le Hôpital Saint-Louis* written by Parisian physicians, A. Hardy and A. Montmeja. The color dramatically draws attention to the raw, eaten away appearance of this patient's face. Lupus was a generic term used to describe any of the conditions in which a patient's face looked as though it had been chewed by a wolf (Latin -lupus). This is a case of superficial and deep tissue infection by tuberculosis. Cutaneous manifestations of tuberculosis were quite common in the pre-antibiotic era and had to be differentiated from syphilis. These 'lupus' patients often wore masks or covered their faces when in public. Because the public could not often identify the difference between the facial deformities caused by tuberculosis from those caused by syphilis, social ostracism became the norm.

Before the development of color photography in the twentieth century, an artist would often hand-color photographs to give them a more realistic look. For scientific purposes, these images seemed more credible. Medical artists, however, at times exaggerated clinical defects to make them more pronounced and memorable. Dermatologists were among the first to produce photographic atlases as their specialty was visually based on observable skin changes. Montmeja became the official photographer for the Hôpital Saint-Louis in Paris. He also worked with other Parisian physicians who wanted to produce photographic texts. Montmeja together and with ophthalmologist, Edouard Meyer, M.D., published the first photographic atlas on eye surgery.

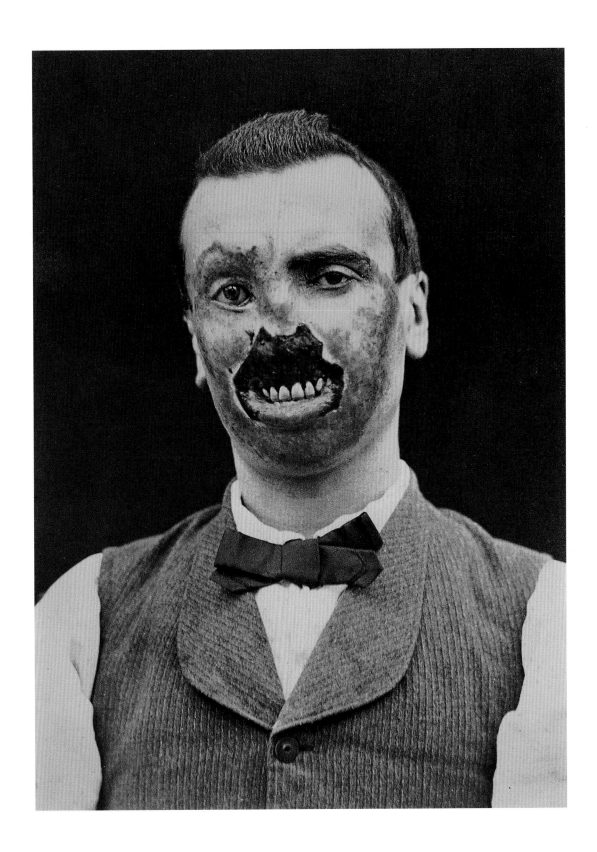

24

Rodent Cancer of the Nose: Invading Nasal Passages

Albumen Print, 3 by 4 inches
London
1865

In the nineteenth century, basal cell carcinoma in the nasal area generally proved fatal. Invariably infection or uncontrollable hemorrhage killed the patient. Numerous photographs have survived from photography's earliest era, documenting the extent of the disease, which fascinated physicians. In the pre-antiseptic era the tolerance of the amount of facial destruction and patient survival is amazing. This photograph documents one of the facially destructive cancers. This woman appears to have one area of her face cleanly cut out. It was actually treated with chemicals by London physician, Charles H. Moore. He published this photograph in one of the first textbooks in medicine (1865) containing photographs. This image of 'Rodent Cancer' was pasted or 'tipped-in' by hand. Dr. Moore's description of the disease is classic. "A disease more repulsive and distressing can hardly be conceived than a rodent cancer of the face. Commencing in some trifling manner in the skin it spreads in all directions, slowly it grows and ulcerates, but never heals." This patient, Mary H., was admitted to Middlesex Hospital after a mole on her nose began to enlarge. Treatment was initiated with the application of 'Donovan's Solution', an unnerving mixture of arsenic, iodine and mercury. Two months later the wound was packed with 'chloride of zinc paste,' which hardened and sloughed away. Although a painful application this remedy occasionally seemed to produce desirable results. Miraculously Mary H.'s cancer disappeared without a trace after a few months. Vulcanite prosthetic masks were often used by these patients in an effort to hide the defect. The open wounds were obviously prone to drainage and infection. Treatment of basal cell carcinoma with caustic agents is still used to this day. However, to assure no disease remains surgical excision with clear margins after pathologic examination is the best therapy.

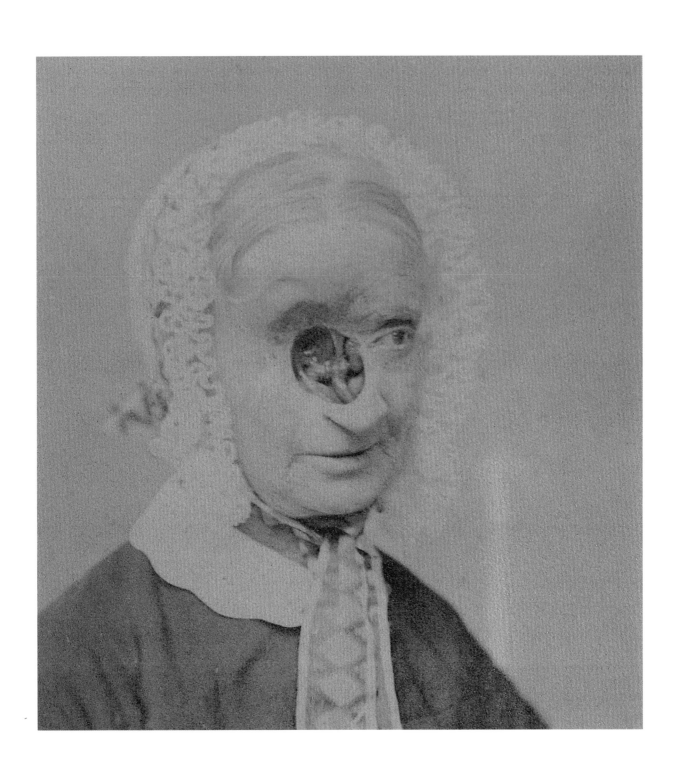

25

Nasal Epithelioma: Syphilis of the Nose Mimicking Carcinoma

Albumen Print, 4 by 5 inches
circa 1870

Accurate diagnosis of respiratory tract disease was difficult prior to the elucidation of the germ theory of disease, and the development of laboratory based medicine in the early twentieth century. The true etiology as to the cause of disease, its progression and treatment were largely unknown. Syphilis was called the 'great mimicker.' It could imitate the signs and symptoms of almost every known disease including cancer. Syphilis was always of grave concern to physicians. The disease was particularly rampant among children who had been infected by parents often in utero. Congenital syphilis often created horrendous deformities including blindness, deafness and horrendous loss of facial features. This case almost fooled physicians because the patient was young with no other apparent signs or symptoms. The 11 year old boy was brought to the surgical clinic of Philadelphia's Jefferson Medical College complaining of a painful growth on his nose. Physicians believed the lesion to be an epithelioma and took biopsies, which appeared to reveal the characteristic features of cancer. However Samuel Weisell Gross, M.D. (1837-1889, the son of the eminent American surgeon Samuel David Gross, M.D. (1805-1884), was an expert on genital disease and had the father of the boy as a patient. Dr. Gross studied the case history and decided he was suffering from syphilis. His mother was never reported to have the disease but his father had both primary and secondary symptoms. Furthermore, although the boy was born healthy and never had a skin eruption, he was afflicted with the 'snuffles', a pathologic sign of syphilis. The treatment instituted by Dr. Gross consisted of the administration of iodide of potassium combined with bichloride of mercury three times in a 24 hour period, then the cleaning of the wound with an emollient poultice. After the crusts had dropped off, the entire surface of the boy's face was treated with acid nitrate of mercury every second day. Within two weeks, the pain associated with the lesion had disappeared and the ulcer was covered with a crusted secretion. This photograph was taken to document the condition and treatment. Several physicians who had examined the boy for the first time during this stage believed he had a malignancy. Dr. Gross, however, stuck to his diagnosis of congenital syphilis and continued the treatments. Three months later the wound was healed and scarred over.

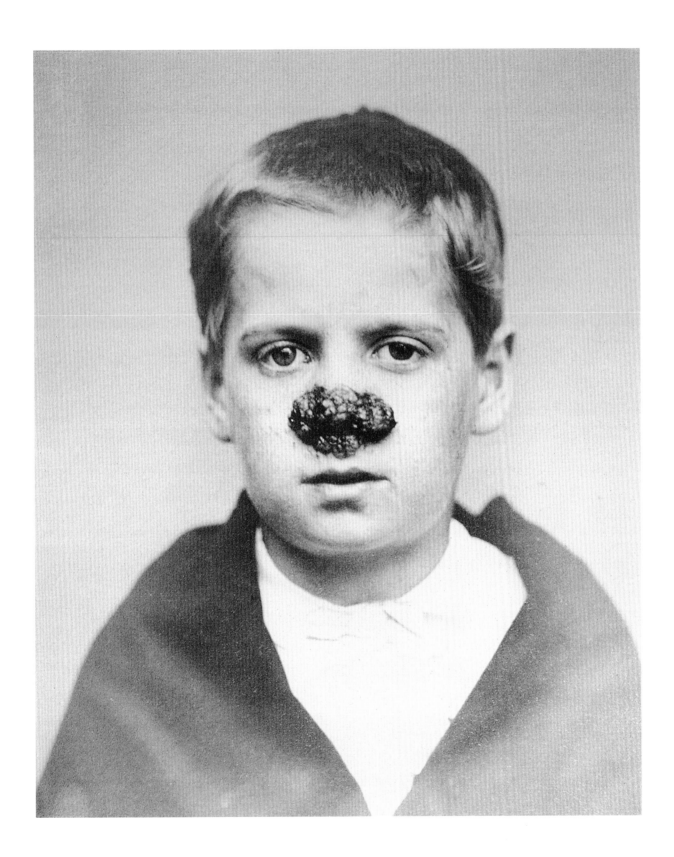

BIBLIOGRAPHY

Adams, George Worthington. *The Medical History of the Union Army in The Civil War*. Henry Schuman: New York, 1952.

Bordley III, James, M.D., and A. McGehee Harvey, M.D. *Two Centuries of American Medicine: 1776-1976*. W.B. Saunders Co.: Philadelphia, Pennsylvania, 1976.

Brandt, Allan M. *No Magic Bullet: A Social History of Venereal Disease in the United States Since 1880*. Oxford University Press: New York, New York, 1985.

Brieger, Gert H. *Medical America in the Nineteenth Century: Readings from the Literature*. Johns Hopkins Press: Baltimore, Maryland, 1972.

Burns, Stanley B., M.D., and Richard Glenner, D.D.S. et al. *The American Dentist: A Pictorial History with a Presentation of Early Dental Photography in America*. Pictorial Histories Publishing Co.: Missoula, MO, 1990.

Burns, Stanley B., M.D., and Ira M. Rutkow, M.D. *American Surgery: An Illustrated History*. Lippincott-Raven Publishers: Philadelphia, PA, 1998.

Burns, Stanley B., M.D. *Early Medical Photography in America: 1839-1883*. The Burns Archive: New York, NY, 1983.

Burns, Stanley B., M.D., and Sherwin Nuland, M.D. et al. *The Face of Mercy: A Photographic History of Medicine at War*. Random House: New York, NY, 1993.

Burns, Stanley B., M.D., and Joel-Peter Witkin, et al. *Harm's Way: Lust & Madness, Murder & Mayhem*. Twin Palms Publishers: Santa Fe, New Mexico, 1994.

Burns, Stanley B., M.D., and Joel-Peter Witkin, et al. *Masterpieces of Medical Photography: Selections From The Burns Archive*. Twelvetrees Press: Pasadena, CA 1987.

Burns, Stanley B., M.D. *A Morning's Work: Medical Photographs from The Burns Archive & Collection 1843-1939*. Twin Palms Publishers: Santa Fe, New Mexico, 1998.

Burns, Stanley B., M.D., and Jacques Gasser, M.D. *Photographie et Médecine 1840-1880*. Insitut universitaire d'histoire de la santé publique: Lausanne, Switzerland, 1991.

Burns, Stanley B., M.D., *Sleeping Beauty: Memorial Photography in America*. TweleveTrees Press: Altadena, California, 1990.

Burns, Stanley B., M.D. and Elizabeth A. Burns. *Sleeping Beauty II: Grief, Bereavement and The Family in Medical Photography, American & European Traditions*. Burns Archive Press: New York, NY, 2002.

Calkins, Alonzo, M.D. *Opium and the Opium Appetite with Notices of Alcoholic Beverages, Cannabis Indica, Tobacco and Coca, and Tea and Coffee, in Their Hygienic Aspects and Pathologic Relations*. J. B. Lippincott & Co.: Philadelphia, Pennsylvania, 1871.

Clarke, Edward H., M.D., et al. *A Century of American Medicine: 1776-1876*. Burt Franklin: New York, New York, 1876.

Cummins, S. Lyle. M.D. *Tuberculosis in History: From the 17th Century to our Times*. Bailliere, Tindall and Cox: London, 1949.

Davis, Loyal. *Fifty Years of Surgical Progress: 1905-1955*. Franklin H. Martin Memorial Foundation: Chicago, Illinois, 1955.

Dieffenbach, William H. *Hydrotherapy: A Brief Therapy of the Practical Value of Water in Disease for Students and Practicians of Medicine*. Rebman Co.: New York, New York, 1909.

Donahue, M. Patricia. *Nursing: The Finest Art*. Mosby: St. Louis, Missouri, 1996.

Duffy, John. *The Healers: A History of American Medicine*. University of Illinois Press: Urbana, Illinois, 1976.

Dubos, Rene and Jean. *The White Plague: Tuberculosis, Man and Society*. Little Brown and Company: Boston, 1952.

Editors. *Harrison's Principles of Internal Medicine, Thirteenth Edition*. McGraw Hill: Health Professionals Division, 1994.

Fee, Elizabeth and Daniel M. Fox. *AIDS: The Burdens of History*. University of California Press: Berkeley, California, 1988.

Frizot , Michel. *The New History of Photography*. Könemann Verlagsgesellschaft mbH, Koln, Germany, 1998.

Fulop-Miller, Rene. *Triumph Over Pain*. The Literary Guild of America: New York, 1938.

Fye, W. Bruce. *The Development of American Physiology: Scientific Medicine in the Nineteenth Century*. Johns Hopkins University Press: Baltimore, Maryland, 1987.

Fye, W. Bruce. *American Cardiology: The History of a Specialty and Its College*. Johns Hopkins University Press: Baltimore, Maryland, 1996.

Garrison, Fielding H., M.D. *An Introduction to the History of Medicine. With Medical Chronology, Suggestions for Study and Bibliographic Data*. W.B. Saunders Co.: Philadelphia, Pennsylvania, 1913.

Gevitz, Norman. *The DO's: Osteopathic Medicine in America*. Johns Hopkins University Press: Baltimore, Maryland, 1982.

Gillett, Mary C. *The Army Medical Department: 1818-1865*. Center of Military History United States Army: Washington, DC, 1987.

Gorin, George, M.D. *History of Ophthalmology*. Publish or Perish, Inc.: Wilmington, Delaware, 1982.

Hechtlinger, Adelaide. *The Great Patent Medicine Era or Without Benefit of Doctor*. Grosset & Dunlap, Inc.: New York, New York, 1970.

Hurwitz, Alfred, M.D. and George Degenshein, M.D. *Milestones in Modern Surgery*. Hoeber-Harper: New York, NY 1958.

Johnson, Stephen L. *The History of Cardiac Surgery: 1896-1955*. Johns Hopkins Press: Baltimore, Maryland, 1970.

Keen, William W., M.D. *Surgery; Its Principles and Practice, by Various Authors*. W.B. Saunders Co., Philadelphia, PA, 1908.

Kelly, Howard & Walter Burrage. *Dictionary of American Medical Biography*. D. Appleton and Co.: New York, 1928.

Kevles, Bettyann Holtzmann. *Naked to the Bone: Medical Imaging in the Twentieth Century*. Helix Books: Addison Wesley, Reading, Massachusetts, 1997.

Kevorkian, Jack, M.D. *The Story of Dissection*. Philosophical Library: New York, New York, 1959.

Kiple, Kenneth F. *The Cambridge World History of Human Disease*. Cambridge University Press: New York, NY, 1993.

Leibowitz, J.O. *The History of Coronary Heart Disease*. Wellcome Institute of the History of Medicine: London, England, 1970.

Levinson, Abraham, M.D. *Pioneers of Pediatrics*. Froben Press: New York, NY, 1936.

Lieberman, Phillip L., M.D., and Michael Blaiss, M.D. *Atlas of Allergic Diseases*. Current Medicine, Inc.: Philadelphia, Pennsylvania, 2002.

Lopate, Carol. *Women in Medicine*. Johns Hopkins Press: Baltimore, Maryland, 1968.

Lyons, Albert S., M.D., and Joseph Petrucelli, II, M.D. *Medicine: An Illustrated History*. Harry N. Abrams, Inc.: New York, NY, 1978.

Margotta, Roberto. *The Story of Medicine*. Golden Press: New York, NY, 1967.

McHenry, Lawrence C., Jr., M.D. *Garrison's History of Neurology*. Charles C. Thomas: Springfield, Illinois, 1969.

Morton, Leslie T. *A Medical Bibliography (Garrison and Morton): An Annotated Check-List of Texts Illustrating the History of Medicine*. Andre Deutsch, Morrison and Gibb, Ltd.: London,1970.

Otis, George A., M.D., et al. *Medical and Surgical History of the War of* the Rebellion, six volumes. Washington D.C., Surgeon General's Office, 1870-1888. Surgical Section, Part I, 1870; Part II, 1876, 1879; Part III, 1888. Medical Section, Part II, 1879.

Packard, Francis R., M.D. History of Medicine in the United States. Hafner Press: New York, NY, 1973.

Parascandola, John, ed. The History of Antibiotics: A Symposium. American Institute of the History of Pharmacy: Madison, Wisconsin, 1980.

Puderbach P. The Massage Operator. Benedict Lust: Butler, New Jersey, 1925.

Pusey, Wm. Allen, M.D. The History of Dermatology. Charles C. Thomas: Springfield, Illinois, 1933.

Reverby, Susan M. Ordered to Care: The Dilemma of American Nursing, 1850-1945. Cambridge University Press: New York, NY 1987.

Rice, Thurman B., M.D. The Conquest of Disease. Macmillian Co.: New York, NY, 1932.

Romm, Sharon., M.D. The Changing Face of Beauty. Mosby Year Book: St. Louis, Missouri, 1992.

Rothstein, William G. American Physicians in the Nineteenth Century: From Sects to Science. Johns Hopkins University Press: Baltimore, Maryland, 1972.

Rowntree, Leonard G., M.D. Amid Masters of Twentieth Century Medicine: A Panorama of Persons and Pictures. Charles C. Thomas: Springfield, Illinois, 1958.

Sarnecky, Mary T., DNSc. A History of the U.S. Army Nurse Corps. University of Pennsylvania Press: Philadelphia, Pennsylvania, 1999.

Schmidt, J.E., M.D. Medical Discoveries: Who and When. Charles C. Thomas: Springfield, Illinois, 1959.

Silverstein, Arthur M., M.D. A History of Immunology. Academic Press, Inc. Harcourt Brace Jovanovich, Publishers: San Diego CA, 1989.

Steiner, Paul E., M.D. Disease in the Civil War: Natural Biological Warfare in 1861-1865. Charles C. Thomas: Springfield, IL, 1968.

Tauber, Alfred and Chernyak. Metchnikoff and the Origins of Immunology: From Metaphor to Theory. Oxford University Press: New York, NY, 1991.

Wallace, Antony F. The Progress of Plastic Surgery: An Introductory History. Willem A. Meeuws: Oxford, England, 1982.

Walker, Kenneth. The Story of Medicine. Oxford University Press: New York, 1955.

Wangensteen, Owen H., M.D. and Sarah D. Wangensteen, The Rise of Surgery: From Empiric Craft to Scientific Discipline. University of Minnesota Press, Minneapolis, 1978.

Weir, Neil. Otolaryngology: An Illustrated History. Butterworths: London, England, 1990.

Welbourn, Richard B., M.D. The History of Endocrine Surgery. Praeger: New York, NY, 1990.

Wershub, Leonard Paul, M.D. Urology: From Antiquity to the 20th Century. Warren H. Green Inc.: St. Louis, Missouri, 1970.

Winslow, Charles-Edward Amory. The Conquest of Epidemic Disease: A Chapter in the History of Ideas. University of Wisconsin Press: Madison, WI, 1943.

Woodward, J.J., M.D. Circular No. 6, Surgeon General's Office: Reports on the Extent and Nature of the Material Available for the Preparation of a Medical and Surgical History of The Rebellion. J.B. Lippincott & Co.: Philadelphia, 1865.

Worden, Gretchen. Mütter Museum of the College of Physicians of Philadelphia. Blast Books: New York, NY, 2002.

Zmijewski, Chester M. and June L. Fletcher. Immunohematology. Appelton-Century-Crofts: Prentice-Hall, New York, NY, 1972.

PHOTOGRAPHIC TERMS

HARD IMAGES

Daguerreotype:
The daguerreotype, the first practical form of photography, was presented to the world in 1839 by Frenchman, Louis J.M. Daguerre. It was popular between 1839-1860. It consisted of an image developed on a polished, silver coated, copper plate. This fragile surface made it necessary to protect the plate behind a glass cover and within a special case. Daguerreotypes and ambrotypes were both produced in standard sizes that had a direct relation to the plate size used in the camera.

Ambrotype:
This form of photography was popular between 1854-1865. The ambrotype was a process using silver sensitive emulsion placed on glass. Like the daguerreotype the surface was fragile and the image was cased.

Tintype:
Although most popular between 1858-1890, tintypes, patented in 1856, were produced as a novelty until about 1940. In the tintype process the silver emulsion was affixed to a thin sheet of iron. This surface was not fragile and tintypes could even be sent through the mail. The term "tintype" comes from the use of tin snips to cut the large sheets of iron.

PAPER PRINTS

The calotype, the first type of paper print made from a paper negative, was invented in 1841. The process was not used in America. In 1851, the collodion wet plate process was developed using glass negatives. The photographic glass negative had to be wet when inserted into the camera and immediately developed while still wet. The paper albumen print was its most popular form. In 1871, Englishman Richard Maddox, MD developed the gelatin based silver print, known as the dry plate process. By the late 1870s instantaneous stop action photographs were possible. Photographs were usually taken by professionals or serious amateurs until 1888 when Kodak introduced roll film with a special camera that allowed anyone to take a photograph. The age of amateur photography began and physicians began to personally document their lives and patients.

Carte de Visite:
Most popular between 1860-1880, the CdV was a $2^1/_4$ by $3^1/_2$ inch paper print pasted onto a card $2^1/_2$ by 4 inches. It was this style photograph that necessitated the creation of the photograph album, so the public could easily compile cards of relatives or celebrities.

Cabinet Card:
Popular between 1875-1895, the cabinet card is a 4 by $5^1/_2$ inch print pasted on a $4^1/_4$ by $6^1/_2$ inch card. Cabinet cards were also assembled in albums.

Stereoview:
Popular from 1850-1930, the stereoview encompassed all the different photographic processes. It consisted of two images each about 3 by $3^1/_2$ taken with a special twin-lens camera. The prints were mounted side by side on a cardboard about $3^1/_2$ by 7 inches. The card was inserted into a stereoscope viewer, which created a 3D effect and gave the viewer the illusion of actually viewing the scene. This three dimensional effect was useful in teaching medical subjects.

Albumen Print:
Popular 1850s-1880, the albumen print was a sharp, detailed paper print produced by the wet plate process. An egg white based emulsion was the key to this process, hence the name 'albumen' print.

Gelatin-Silver Print & other Silver Print Processes:
Popular in various forms from 1880 to today.

Dedication

Many physicians who treated and investigated tuberculosis contracted and succumbed to the disease. The list is voluminous and contains many medical luminaries including Dr. Rene Laënnec, inventor of the stethoscope. The sacrifices made by physicians for the advancement of medicine are legendary. Those who died or were mutilated in the development of radiology are well known but the specialists and conquerors fighting tuberculosis have never been fully appreciated. To these selfless individuals, I dedicate this work.

Acknowledgements

First and foremost I would like to thank my family who are integral parts of the Burns Archive. They have assisted me, tirelessly, in preparing this historic compilation. My wife, Sara, helps with collecting, cataloging and archiving the collection, and directs the stock photography use of the material. More importantly she serves as my sounding board and editor helping to clarify my ideas. My daughter, Elizabeth, designed and directed the entire production of these volumes from their conception to the final product.

I am most grateful to Saul G. Hornik, MS, RPh, medical marketing consultant. It was his enthusiasm and recognition of the educational importance of my medical, photographic collection, together with his tireless work that made this publication a reality. I give my thanks to Eric Malter, President of MD Communications, for his support of this project. I also wish to express my sincere appreciation to Christopher J. Carney, Director of Training Services of GlaxoSmithKline for understanding the educational value in using the visual history of the past as a foundation for the future.

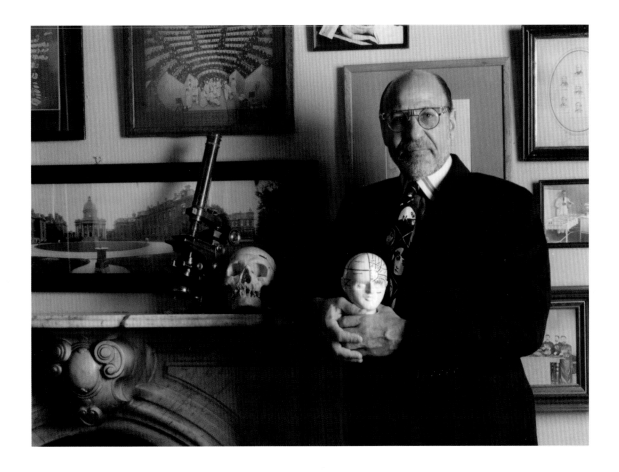

STANLEY B. BURNS, M.D., F.A.C.S.

Stanley B. Burns, M.D., F.A.C.S., a practicing New York City ophthalmic surgeon, is also an internationally distinguished photographic historian, author, curator and collector. His collection, started in 1975, is considered to be the most comprehensive private, early, historic photograph collection in the world. Contained within this archive of over 700,000 vintage prints is the finest and most comprehensive compilation of early medical photographs, consisting of 50,000 images taken between 1840 and 1940. These medical photographs have been showcased in countless publications films and museum exhibitions. France's Channel Plus prepared a documentary on his work as part of the *Great Collectors of the World Series*. Dr. Burns has been an active medical historian since 1970. From 1979-81, he was President of the Medical Archivist of New York State. He has been a member of the medical history departments of The Albert Einstein College of Medicine and The State University of New York, Medical College at Stony Brook; Curator of photographic archives at both The Israeli Institute on The History of Medicine (1978-1993) and The Museum of The Foundation of The American Academy of Ophthalmology. Currently, he is a contributing editor for five specialty medical journals. The Burns Archive, his stock photography and publishing entity, is a valuable photographic resource for both researchers and the media. Using his unique collection Dr. Burns has written ten award winning photo-history books, hundreds of articles and curated dozens of exhibitions. His film company, Black Mirror Films, produced *Death in America*, an award willing documentary on the history of death practices in America. He is currently working on several medical exhibitions and books, as well as photographic history books on criminology, Judaica, Germans in WW II and African Americans. He can be reached through his web site www.burnsarchive.com.

OTHER BOOKS

Sleeping Beauty II: Grief, Bereavement and The Family in Memorial Photography, American & European Traditions

A Mornings Work: Medical Photographs from The Burns Archive & Collection, 1843-1939

Forgotten Marriage: The Painted Tintype & The Decorative Frame 1860-1910, A Lost Chapter in American Portraiture

American Surgery: An Illustrated History
co-author: Ira M. Rutkow, M.D.

Harm's Way: Lust & Madness, Murder & Mayhem
co-authors: Joel-Peter Witkin, et al

The Face of Mercy: A Photographic History of Medicine at War
co-authors: Matthew Naythons, M.D. and Sherwin Nuland, M.D.

Photographie et Médecine 1840-1880
co-author: Jacques Gasser, M.D.

Sleeping Beauty: Memorial Photography in America

The American Dentist: A Pictorial History
co-authors: Richard Glenner, D.D.S. and Audrey Davis, PhD.

Masterpieces of Medical Photography: Selections From The Burns Archive
co-author: Joel-Peter Witkin

Early Medical Photography in America: 1839-1883

THE BURNS ARCHIVE PRESS
140 EAST 38TH STREET • NEW YORK, N.Y. 10016
TEL: 212-889-1938 • FAX: 212-481-9113 • WWW.BURNSARCHIVE.COM